Table of Contents

Introduction

With the ever popularity of processed foods coupled with the rising need of individuals to do things instantly, people have succumbed to consuming more fast food and instant food than ever. This has led to people suffering from weight gain and other metabolic diseases like diabetes, high blood pressure, stroke and many others.

While modern medicine makes it possible to treat symptoms of diseases caused by a bad diet, wouldn't it be better to stop the progression of any diseases by eating the right foods? Although eating the right food is ideal, the problem is that most people tend to become dissuaded to eating healthy because the act of preparing meals is already taxing enough.

But eating the right and healthy foods is not so hard as everyone thinks. The secret to eating healthy is to spend less time with meal preparations by using a crockpot. Thus, this book will serve as your guide on how to prepare delicious yet easy-to-prepare ketogenic crockpot meals.

Chapter 1: Crockpot Uses, Tips and Tricks

The crockpot or slow cooker is a countertop kitchen appliance that cooks food at low temperature. Thus, this allows you to prepare your food hours before you actually eat them. Crockpots are used in cooking not only soups and stews but also other types of foods such as casseroles, roasts, and desserts.

Using the crockpot is very simple. All there is to it is to put the ingredients and select the cooking setting so that it starts cooking the food slowly. This nifty kitchen appliance cooks food at temperature ranges between 71°C and 74°C. The crockpot has a heating element that creates a steady temperature that cooks food for longer. The lid is also airtight so it forms condensation that allows effective transfer of heat within the crockpot. This is also the reason why crockpots do not require a lot of liquid to cook food. And since food is cooked below the boiling point thus it can retain all the healthy enzymes and nutrients in the food.

Using the Crockpot

As popular kitchen appliances, crockpots are very beneficial as they are better in cooking cheaper and tougher meat cuts. Moreover, since the food is cooked at low temperature, it does not burn the food at all thus retaining the rich flavor of the food. But how do you cook the crockpot? Below are effective cooking tips when using crockpots.

- Fill the crockpot with ½ or ¾ of liquid as too much liquid will require a longer time to heat up the food thus you might need extra hours to completely cook your food.
- Foods that are placed at the bottom will cook faster and moister because they will be immersed in the liquid. Place root vegetables or meat at the bottom for a delicious meal.
- Remove the skin and trim extra fat as it will melt while cooking. This will also cook the food too quickly.

- Never lift the lid to check the status of your food. The thing is that every time you lift the lid, you lose necessary heat to cook your food so you need to extend the cooking time to 20 more minutes.

Tips and Tricks

You can cook different types of food in the crockpot so there are specific tips that you need to know in order to effectively cook any kinds of food with your crockpot. Below are great tips and tricks when cooking food in a crockpot.

- Cook all ground meats in a skillet first to drain all fats before cooking. This will also make the meat more flavorful and also remove the fat that can affect the cooking time.
- When cooking seafood, add them during the last hour of cooking time as cooking it for longer can cause them to have a rubbery texture.
- Brown large pieces of meat in a skillet before cooking in the crockpot to create additional flavor.
- Add tender vegetables at the last 45 minutes of cooking time so that they don't get overcooked.
- Dairy products particularly milk and cream should be added last. Overcooking the dairy products leads to curdling or the separation of protein of the milk from its natural water content.

Eggs with Spinach and Yogurt

Serves: 4
Cook Time: 3 hours

Ingredients

- 1 clove of garlic, minced
- 2/3 cup plain Greek yogurt
- 2 tablespoons grass-fed butter, unsalted
- 4 large eggs, beaten
- 1 teaspoon fresh oregano, chopped
- Salt and pepper to taste
- 2 tablespoons olive oil
- 10 cups fresh spinach, chopped
- ¼ teaspoon red pepper flakes, crushed
- 2 tablespoon scallions, chopped

Instructions

1. In a mixing bowl, combine garlic, yogurt, butter, and eggs. Stir in oregano and season with salt and pepper to taste.
2. Grease the bottom of the CrockPot with olive oil.
3. Arrange the spinach and pour over the egg mixture.
4. Sprinkle with pepper flakes and scallions on top.
5. Close the lid and cook on high for 2 hours or on low for 3 hours.

Nutrition information: Calories per serving: 247; Carbohydrates: 6.8g; Protein: 17.8g; Fat: 21.4g; Sugar: 0g; Sodium: 410mg; Fiber: 3.5g

Cowboy Breakfast Casserole

Serves: 6
Cook Time: 3 hours

Ingredients

- 1-pound ground beef
- 5 eggs, beaten
- 1 cup grass-fed Monterey Jack cheese, shredded
- Salt and pepper to taste
- 1 avocado, peeled and diced
- A handful of cilantro, chopped
- A dash of hot sauce

Instructions

1. In a skillet over medium flame, sauté the beef for three minutes until slightly golden.
2. Pour into the CrockPot and pour in eggs.
3. Sprinkle with cheese on top and season with salt and pepper to taste.
4. Close the lid and cook on high for 4 hours or on low for 6 hours.
5. Serve with avocado, cilantro and hot sauce.

Nutrition information: Calories per serving: 439; Carbohydrates: 4.5g; Protein: 32.7g; Fat: 31.9g; Sugar: 0g; Sodium: 619mg; Fiber: 1.8g

Eggs and Vegetables Omelet

Serves: 4
Cook Time: 3 hours

Ingredients

- 2 tablespoons coconut oil
- 4 eggs, beaten
- 1 cup spinach, chopped
- ½ cup cauliflower, chopped
- ½ cup broccoli, chopped
- 1 cup grass-fed sharp cheddar cheese, shredded
- Salt and pepper to taste

Instructions

1. Grease the inside of the CrockPot with coconut oil.
2. Pour in eggs, spinach, cauliflower, and broccoli. Stir to combine.
3. Add in the cheese and season with salt and pepper to taste.
4. Close the lid and cook on high for 2 hours or on low for 3 hours.

Nutrition information: Calories per serving: 257; Carbohydrates: 3.4g; Protein: 13.2g; Fat: 21.5g; Sugar: 0g; Sodium: 319mg; Fiber:2.7 g

Broccoli Egg Casserole

Serves: 5
Cook Time: 3 hours

Ingredients
- 4 eggs, beaten
- ½ cup full-fat milk
- 3 tablespoons grass-fed butter, melted
- 1 ½ cup broccoli florets, chopped
- Salt and pepper to taste

Instructions
1. Beat the eggs and milk in a mixing bowl.
2. Grease the bottom of the CrockPot with melted butter.
3. Add in the broccoli florets in the CrockPot and pour the egg mixture.
4. Season with salt and pepper to taste.
5. Close the lid and cook on high for 2 hours or on low for 3 hours.

Nutrition information: Calories per serving: 217; Carbohydrates:4.6 g; Protein: 11.6g; Fat: 16.5g; Sugar: 0.7g; Sodium: 674mg; Fiber: 2.3g

Spinach, Goat Cheese and Beef Omelet

Serves: 2
Cook Time: 3 hours

Ingredients
- 4 ounces ground beef
- 2 cloves of garlic, minced
- ½ tablespoon butter
- 4 eggs, beaten
- 2 ounces organic fresh goat cheese
- 2 cups baby spinach leaves, rinsed and drained
- Salt and pepper to taste
- 1 avocado, sliced
- ½ cup tomatoes, chopped

Instructions
1. Heat skillet over medium high flame and sauté the beef and garlic until all sides turn light golden brown. Turn off the flame and add in the butter.
2. Pour into the CrockPot and add the eggs.
3. Stir in the goat cheese and spinach leaves.
4. Season with salt and pepper to taste.
5. Close the lid and cook on high for 4 hours or on low for 5 hours until the beef is cooked.
6. Serve with avocado slices and tomatoes.

Nutrition information: Calories per serving: 368; Carbohydrates: 8.2g; Protein: 22.9g; Fat: 26.7g; Sugar: 2.1g; Sodium: 736mg; Fiber: 4.8g

Roasted Tomato Shakshuka

Serves: 5
Cook Time: 4 hours

Ingredients

- 1 onion, chopped
- 1 bell pepper, seeded and chopped
- 1 ½ pounds cherry tomatoes
- ½ tablespoon cumin seeds
- 2 sprigs thyme leaves
- ¼ cup extra virgin olive oil
- 4 organic eggs
- Salt and pepper to taste
- 1 tablespoon parsley, chopped
- A pinch of cayenne pepper

Instructions

1. Place the onions, bell pepper, cherry tomatoes, cumin and thyme leaves in the food processor. Pulse until smooth.
2. Pour half of the olive oil in the CrockPot and pour the tomato mixture.
3. Break gently the eggs on top of the tomato mixture.
4. Season with salt and pepper to taste.
5. Close the lid and cook on high for 3 hours or on low for 4 hours.
6. An hour before the cooking time ends, pour in the remaining oil and sprinkle with parsley and cayenne pepper.
7. Close the lid and continue cooking for another hour or two.

Nutrition information: Calories per serving: 253; Carbohydrates: 9.5g; Protein: 27.5g; Fat: 12.8g; Sugar: 1.4g; Sodium: 371mg; Fiber: 4.7g

CrockPot Fisherman's Eggs

Serves: 2
Cook Time: 3 hours

Ingredients

- 1 can organic sardines in olive oil
- 2 organic eggs
- ½ cup arugula, rinsed and drained
- ½ of artichoke hearts, chopped
- Salt and pepper to taste

Instructions

1. Put the sardines in the bottom of the CrockPot.
2. Break the eggs on top of the sardines and add the arugula and artichokes on top.
3. Season with salt and pepper to taste.
4. Close the lid and cook on high for 2 hours or on low for 3 hours.

Nutrition information: Calories per serving:315; Carbohydrates: 3.5g; Protein: 28g; Fat:20.6 g; Sugar: 0g; Sodium: 491mg; Fiber: 1.3g

Green Buttered Eggs

Serves: 2
Cook Time: 3 hours

Ingredients

- 2 tablespoons organic grass-fed butter
- 1 tablespoon coconut oil
- 2 cloves of garlic, chopped
- ½ cup cilantro, chopped
- 1 teaspoon thyme leaves
- 4 organic eggs, beaten
- ¼ teaspoon cayenne pepper
- Salt and pepper to taste

Instructions

1. Place butter and coconut oil in a skillet heated over medium flame.
2. Add in the garlic and sauté until fragrant.
3. Add in the cilantro and thyme leaves. Continue stirring until crisp.
4. Pour into the CrockPot and add in the beaten eggs.
5. Season with cayenne pepper, salt and black pepper to taste.
6. Close the lid and cook on high for 2 hours and on low for 3 hours.

Nutrition information: Calories per serving:311; Carbohydrates: 2.5g; Protein: 14.6g; Fat: g27.5 Sugar:0 g; Sodium: 362mg; Fiber: 1g

Santa Fe's Frittata

Serves: 12
Cook Time: 4 hours

Ingredients

- 10 organic eggs
- ½ cup milk
- Salt and pepper to taste
- 8 ounces ground pork
- 2 cups red and yellow sweet peppers, diced
- ½ cup pepper jack cheese

Instructions

1. Beat eggs and milk in a mixing bowl. Season with salt and pepper to taste. Set aside.
2. Heat a skillet over medium high flame and sauté the ground pork until lightly golden.
3. Pour into the CrockPot and add in the sweet peppers.
4. Pour in the egg mixture and sprinkle cheese on top.
5. Close the lid and cook on high for 3 hours or on low for 4 hours.

Nutrition information: Calories per serving: 169; Carbohydrates: 2.8g; Protein: 11.2g; Fat:11.9 g; Sugar: 0g; Sodium: 269mg; Fiber: 0.5g

Omelet with Olives and Avocado

Serves: 5
Cook Time: 3 hours

Ingredients

- 4 organic eggs
- 2 ounces organic Brie cheese
- ½ teaspoon rosemary, dried
- ½ teaspoon oregano, dried
- 2 tablespoons coconut oil
- 2 tablespoons grass-fed butter
- ½ teaspoon salt
- 10 black olives, pitted and sliced
- 1 avocado, sliced

Instructions

1. In a mixing bowl, combine the eggs, cheese, rosemary, oregano, coconut oil, and butter. Season with salt to taste.
2. Place in the CrockPot and add in the sliced olives.
3. Close the lid and cook on high for 2 hours or on low for 3 hours.
4. Serve with avocado slices.

Nutrition information: Calories per serving:313; Carbohydrates: 2.4g; Protein: 9g; Fat: 30g; Sugar: 0g; Sodium: 372mg; Fiber: 1.2g

Breakfast Lasagna

Serves: 10
Cook Time: 4-5 hours

Ingredients:

- 1 small onion, diced
- 10 ounces lean ground beef
- 2 garlic cloves, minced
- 2 tablespoons olive oil
- ½ teaspoon sea salt
- 6 large eggs
- 1 cup ricotta cheese
- 1 cup mozzarella cheese, grated
- 1 cup feta cheese
- 2 cups spinach, fresh chopped
- 2 medium eggplants, cut into ½-inch slices
- 1 large zucchini, cut into ½-inch slices
- 1 cup marinara sauce, no-sugar-added

Directions: Brown the ground beef, garlic, and onion in a frying pan over medium-heat; add in the marinara sauce and salt, then set aside. Peel the eggplant and zucchini, cut into ½-inch slices. In a mixing bowl, beat the eggs. Grease Crock-Pot with oil. Place the eggplant and zucchini along with spinach in Crock-Pot. Spoon a layer of meat sauce onto veggies. Sprinkle with some mozzarella, feta, and ricotta cheese. Repeat with the veggie layer, meat sauce, cheese and beaten eggs. Finish by topping with some more cheese. Cover and cook on LOW for 4-5 hours and serve warm.

Nutrition Values: Calories: 537, Total Fat: 46 g, Saturated Fat: 19.6 g, Net Carbs: 11.4 g, Dietary Fiber: 5.4 g, Protein: 33 g

Roasted Red Pepper & Kale Omelet

Total Cooking Time: 2-3 hours

Servings: 8

Ingredients:

- ¼ cup green onion, sliced
- 1 cup feta cheese, crumbled
- 2 tablespoons olive oil
- 6 ounces red pepper, diced
- 5 ounces baby kale, chopped
- 10 large eggs
- Black pepper, fresh-ground, to taste
- ½ teaspoon sea salt

Directions:

Spray the inside of Crock-Pot with non-stick cooking spray. In a pan, heat 1 tablespoon of olive oil and sauté the kale until it is softened. Add diced red pepper, onions, and sautéed kale to Crock-Pot. In a mixing bowl, beat the eggs with salt and pepper, adding in the remaining olive oil, and pour over veggie layer. Sprinkle top with crumbled feta cheese. Cover and cook on LOW for 2-3 hours or until the frittata is set. Serve hot.

Nutrition Values:

Calories: 298, Total Fat: 24.4 g, Saturated Fat: 23.4 g, Net Carbs: 3 g, Dietary Fiber: 1.3 g, Protein: 39.4 g

Cheesy Sausage Casserole

Total Cooking Time: **4-5 hours**

Servings: **6-8**

Ingredients:

- 1 ½ cups cheddar cheese, shredded
- ½ cup mayonnaise
- 2 cups green cabbage, shredded
- 2 cups zucchini, diced
- ½ cup onion, diced
- 8 large eggs
- 1 lb. pork sausage
- 1 teaspoon sage, ground, dried
- 2 teaspoons prepared yellow mustard
- Cayenne pepper to taste
- ¼ teaspoon sea salt
- ¼ teaspoon black pepper

Directions:

Using cooking spray, grease the inside of the Crock-Pot. In a mixing bowl, whisk together eggs, mayonnaise, cheese, mustard, dried ground sage, cayenne pepper, salt, and black pepper. Layer half of the sausage, cabbage, zucchini, and onions into the Crock-Pot. Repeat with the remaining ingredients of zucchini, onion, sausage and cabbage. Pour the egg mixture onto the layered ingredients. Cook for 4-5 hours on LOW, until it is golden brown on the edges and set. Serve warm.

Nutritional Values:

Calories: 484, Total Fat: 38.85 g, Saturated Fat: 21.6 g, Net Carbs: 6.39 g, Dietary Fiber: 1.8 g, Protein: 26.4 g

Crock-Pot Veggie Omelet

Total Cooking Time: **2 hours**

Servings: **4**

Ingredients:

- 6 large eggs
- 4 cups spinach, fresh, chopped
- 1 ½ cups white mushrooms, sliced
- 2 cloves garlic, crushed
- 1 cup feta cheese, crumbled
- 2 tablespoons of coconut oil
- Salt and pepper to taste

Directions:

Heat the coconut oil in Crock-Pot. Set aside. In a mixing bowl, combine garlic, eggs, salt, and pepper. Add mushrooms and spinach to the mix. Cover and cook for about 2 hours, or until omelet is set. Check it at about 1 hour and 15 minutes into cooking time. When the omelet is cooked, add the feta and fold in half. Transfer to serving plate.

Nutritional Values:

Calories: 659, Total Fat: 55.5 g, Saturated Fat: 30.3 g, Net Carbs: 7.7 g, Dietary Fiber: 2.8 g, Protein: 30.9 g

Crock-Pot Breakfast Casserole

Total Cooking Time: 10-12 hours

Servings: 8

Ingredients:

- 1 lb. ground sausage, cooked, drained
- 12-ounce package bacon slices, crumbled, cooked, drained
- 1 dozen eggs
- 1 cup heavy white cream
- ½ cup feta cheese, chopped
- 1 teaspoon sea salt
- 1 teaspoon black pepper
- 2 cups Monterrey Jack cheese, shredded
- 1 ½ cups spinach, fresh
- 1 ½ cups mushrooms, fresh, sliced
- 1 green bell pepper, diced
- 1 medium sweet yellow onion, diced
- 4 cups daikon radish hashed browns

Directions:

Place a layer of hashed browns on bottom of Crock-Pot. Follow with a layer of sausage and bacon, then add onions, spinach, green pepper, mushrooms and cheese. In a mixing bowl, beat the eggs, cream, salt, and pepper together. Pour over mixture in Crock-Pot. Cover and cook on LOW for 10-12 hours.

Nutritional Values:

Calories: 443.6, Carbohydrates: 8 g, Fiber: 1.95 g, Net Carbohydrates: 6.05 g, Protein: 18.1 g, Fat: 38.25 g

"Baked" Creamy Brussels Sprouts

Total Cooking Time: 2 hours and 25 minutes

Servings: 2 (serving size is ½ of recipe—6.3 ounces)

Ingredients:

- 14 Brussels sprouts
- ¼ cup Parmesan cheese, grated
- 2 garlic cloves
- ½ cup cream cheese
- 2 tablespoons extra virgin olive oil
- 1 teaspoon balsamic vinegar
- Salt and pepper to taste

Directions:

Rinse the Brussels sprouts in cold water to remove dirt and dust. Discard the first leaves. Pour oil into Crock-Pot and add Brussels sprouts. Add in the remaining ingredients and stir. Cover and cook for 3-4 hours on low or 1-2 hours on HIGH. Before serving, sprinkle with Parmesan or feta cheese. Let cheese melt for 2 or 3 minutes.

Nutrition Values:

Calories: 228.7, Total Fat: 15.85 g, Saturated Fat: 8.95 g, Cholesterol: 49.28 mg, Sodium: 332.45 mg, Potassium: 522.11 mg, Total Carbohydrates: 8.57 g, Sugar: 4.16 g, Protein: 10.93 g

Chive & Bacon Muffins

Total Cooking Time: 2 hours and 15 minutes

Servings: 12 (serving size: 3.5 ounces)

Ingredients:

- 2 cups almond flour
- 6 slices bacon
- 2 teaspoons baking powder
- 1 ½ teaspoons garlic powder
- ¼ teaspoon sea salt
- ½ cup olive oil
- ¾ cup milk
- 1 egg, beaten
- 1 1/3 cup Parmesan cheese, grated
- 4 teaspoons chives, dried

Directions:

Place the bacon on a micro-wave safe plate. Heat the bacon in the micro-wave on high for 4 to 6 minutes. Let it cool and crumble it. In a mixing bowl, combine garlic powder, baking powder, almond flour, chives, cheese, and crumbled bacon. In a different bowl, combine the milk, egg, and olive oil. Combine the dry ingredients with the wet and mix well. Lightly grease muffin pan. Pour batter in muffin cups (fill 3/4 of each muffin cup). Place a trivet in the bottom of Crock-Pot. Place muffin tray on trivet and cover and cook on HIGH for 2 hours. Serve hot or cold.

Nutrition Values:

Calories: 229.83, Total Fat: 214 g, Saturated Fat: 6.34 g, Cholesterol: 39.42 mg, Sodium: 471.34 mg, Potassium: 86.37 mg, Total Carbohydrates: 1.85 g, Fiber: 0.04 g. Sugar: 0.9 g. Protein: 7.58 g

Breakfast Sausage & Cauliflower

Total Cooking Time: 7 hours and 15 minutes

Servings: 6 (serving size is 6.2 ounces)

Ingredients:

- 10 eggs
- 1 lb. breakfast sausage, chopped
- 1 head cauliflower, shredded
- ½ teaspoon mustard
- ¼ cup milk
- 1 ½ cups cheddar cheese, shredded
- Salt and pepper to taste
- Olive oil

Directions:

Whisk together milk, mustard, eggs, salt, and pepper in a mixing bowl. Grease Crock-Pot with olive oil. Place one layer of sausage on the bottom, then cheese, and season with salt and pepper. Repeat layer. Pour egg mixture over all ingredients. Cover and cook on LOW for 6-7 hours or until eggs are set. Serve hot.

Nutrition Values:

Calories: 324.42, Total Fat: 18.01 g, Saturated Fat: 6.96 g, Cholesterol: 259.93 mg, Sodium: 988.86 mg, Potassium: 222.34 mg, Total Carbohydrates: 7.23 g, Fiber: 3.08 g, Sugar: 1.77 g, Protein: 32.48 g

Bacon, Cheese & Spinach Breakfast

Total Cooking Time: 2 hours and 5 minutes

Servings: 6 (5.9 ounces per serving)

Ingredients:

- 1 cup baby spinach, packed
- 6 organic eggs
- 1 cup Parmesan cheese, shredded
- ½ cup cheddar cheese, shredded
- 1/3 cup mushrooms, fresh, diced
- ½ teaspoon garlic powder
- ½ teaspoon onion powder
- ½ teaspoon thyme
- 1 cup plain yogurt
- 1 cup bacon, cooked, crumbled
- Salt and pepper to taste
- Olive oil

Directions:

In a bowl, whisk together dry herbs, salt, pepper, and eggs. Stir in crumbled bacon, shredded cheese, and spinach. Grease the bottom of Crock-Pot with olive oil. Pour the eggs mixture into Crock-Pot, cover and cook on HIGH for about 2 hours. Serve hot.

Nutrition Values:

Calories: 225.6 , Total Fat: 13.9 g, Saturated Fat: 7.15 g, Cholesterol: 215.12 mg, Sodium: 434.51 mg, Potassium: 294.32 mg, Total Carbohydrates: 6.91 g, Fiber: 0.87 g, Sugar: 4.32 g, Protein: 18.44 g

Kale & Feta Breakfast Frittata

Total Cooking Time: 3 hours and 5 minutes

Servings: 6 (4.8 ounces per serving)

Ingredients:

- 2 cups kale, chopped
- ½ cup feta, crumbled
- 2 teaspoons olive oil
- Salt and pepper to taste
- 3 green onions, chopped
- 1 large green pepper, diced
- 8 eggs

Directions:

Heat the olive oil in Crock-Pot and sauté the kale, diced pepper, and chopped green onion for about 2-3 minutes. Beat the eggs in a mixing bowl, pour over other ingredients, and stir. Add salt and pepper and sprinkle crumbled feta cheese on top. Cover and cook on LOW for 2-3 hours, or until the cheese has melted. Serve hot.

Nutrition Values:

Calories: 160.1, Total Fat: 10.71 g, Saturated Fat: 4.2 g, Cholesterol: 259.13 mg, Sodium: 245.78 mg, Potassium: 263.49 mg, Total Carbohydrates: 4.92 g, Fiber: 1.06 g, Sugar: 1.52 g, Protein: 11.24 g

Mustard Garlic Shrimps

Serves: 4
Preparation time: 5 minutes
Cooking time: 2 hours and 30 minutes

Ingredients

- 1 teaspoon olive oil
- 3 tablespoons garlic, minced
- 1-pound shrimp, shelled and deveined
- 1 teaspoon Dijon mustards
- Salt and pepper to taste
- Parsley for garnish

Instructions

1. In a skillet, heat the olive oil and sauté the garlic until fragrant and slightly browned. Transfer to the crockpot and place the shrimps and Dijon mustard. Stir to combine.
2. Season with salt and pepper to taste.
3. Close the lid and cook on low for 2 hours or high for 30 minutes.
4. Once done, sprinkle with parsley.

Nutrition information: Calories per serving: 138; Carbohydrates: 3.2g; Protein: 23.8g; Fat: 2.7g; Sugar: 0.5g; Sodium: 535mg; Fiber: 0.9g

Mustard-Crusted Salmon

Serves: 4
Preparation time: 3 minutes
Cooking time: 4 hours

Ingredients

- 4 pieces salmon fillets
- salt and pepper to taste
- 2 teaspoons lemon juice
- 2 tablespoons stone-ground mustard
- ¼ cup full sour cream

Instructions

1. Season salmon fillets with salt and pepper to taste. Sprinkle with lemon juice.
2. Rub the stone-ground mustard all over the fillets.
3. Place inside the crockpot and cook on high for 2 hours or on low for 4 hours.
4. An hour before the cooking time, pour in the sour cream on top of the fish.
5. Continue cooking until the fish becomes flaky.

Nutrition information: Calories per serving: 74; Carbohydrates: 4.2g; Protein: 25.9g; Fat:13.8 g; Sugar: 1.3g; Sodium: 536mg; Fiber: 2.5g

Five-Spice Tilapia

Serves: 4
Preparation time: 3 minutes
Cooking time: 5 hours

Ingredients
- 4 tilapia fillets
- 1 teaspoon Chinese five-spice powder
- 1 tablespoon sesame oil
- ¼ cup gluten-free soy sauce
- 3 scallions, thinly sliced

Instructions
1. Season the tilapia fillets with the Chinese five-spice powder.
2. Place sesame oil in the crockpot and arrange the fish on top.
3. Cook on high for 2 hours and on low for 4 hours.
4. Halfway through the cooking time, flip the fish to slightly brown the other side.
5. Once cooking time is done, add the soy sauce and scallion and continue cooking for another hour.

Nutrition information: Calories per serving: 153; Carbohydrates: 0.9g; Protein: 25.8g; Fat: 5.6g; Sugar: 0g; Sodium: 424mg; Fiber: 0g

Prosciutto-Wrapped Scallops

Serves: 4
Preparation time: 3 minutes
Cooking time: 3 hours

Ingredients
- 12 large scallops, rinsed and patted dry
- Salt and pepper to taste
- 1 ¼ ounces prosciutto, cut into 12 long strips
- 1 tablespoon extra-virgin olive oil
- 1 tablespoon lemon juice

Instructions
1. Sprinkle individual scallops with salt and pepper to taste.
2. Wrap a prosciutto around the scallops. Set aside.
3. Add oil in crockpot and arrange on top the bacon-wrapped scallops.
4. Pour over the lemon juice.
5. Cook on low for 1 hour or on high for 3 hours.
6. Halfway through the cooking time, flip the scallops.
7. Continue cooking until scallops are done.

Nutrition information: Calories per serving: 113; Carbohydrates: 5g; Protein: 15.9g; Fat:8 g; Sugar:0 g; Sodium: 424mg; Fiber: 3.2g

Express Shrimps and Sausage Jambalaya Stew

Serves: 4
Preparation time: 5 minutes
Cooking time: 3 hours

Ingredients
- 1 teaspoon canola oil
- 8 ounces andouille sausage, cut into slices
- 1 16-ounce bag frozen bell pepper and onion mix
- 1 can chicken broth
- 8 ounces shrimps, shelled and deveined

Instructions
1. In a skillet, heat the oil and sauté the sausages until the sausages have rendered their fat. Set aside.
2. Pour the vegetable mix into the crockpot.
3. Add in the sausages and pour the chicken broth.
4. Stir in the shrimps last.
5. Cook on low for 1 hour or on low for 3 hours.

Nutrition information: Calories per serving: 316; Carbohydrates: 6.3; Protein: 32.1g; Fat: 25.6g; Sugar:0.2 g; Sodium: 425mg; Fiber: 3.2g

Spicy Basil Shrimp

Serves: 4
Preparation time: 3 minutes
Cooking time: 2 hours

Ingredients
- 1-pound raw shrimp, shelled and deveined
- Salt and pepper to taste
- 1 tablespoon butter
- ¼ cup packed fresh basil leaves
- ¼ teaspoon cayenne pepper

Instructions
1. Add all ingredients in the crockpot.
2. Give a stir.
3. Close the lid and cook on high for 30 minutes or on low for 2 hours.
Nutrition information: Calories per serving: 144; Carbohydrates: 1.4g; Protein: 23.4g; Fat: 6.2g; Sugar: 0g; Sodium: 126mg; Fiber:0.5 g

Scallops with Sour Cream and Dill

Serves: 4
Preparation time: 3 minutes
Cooking time: 2 hours

Ingredients

- 1 ¼ pounds scallops
- Salt and pepper to taste
- 3 teaspoons butter
- ¼ cup sour cream
- 1 tablespoon fresh dill

Instructions

1. Add all ingredients into the crockpot.
2. Give a good stir to combine everything.
3. Close the lid and cook on high for 30 minutes or on low for 2 hours.

Nutrition information: Calories per serving: 152; Carbohydrates: 4.3g; Protein: 18.2g; Fat: 5.7g; Sugar: 0.5g; Sodium: 231mg; Fiber: 2.3g

Salmon with Lime Butter

Serves: 4
Preparation time: 3 minutes
Cooking time: 4 hours

Ingredients

- 1-pound salmon fillet cut into 4 portions
- 1 tablespoon butter, melted
- Salt and pepper to taste
- 2 tablespoons lime juice
- ½ teaspoon lime zest, grated

Instructions

1. Add all ingredients in the crockpot.
2. Close the lid.
3. Cook on high for 2 hours and on low for 4 hours.

Nutrition information: Calories per serving: 206; Carbohydrates: 1.8g; Protein:23.7 g; Fat: 15.2g; Sugar: 0g; Sodium:235 mg; Fiber: 0.5g

Chili-Rubbed Tilapia

Serves: 4
Preparation time: 35 minutes
Cooking time: 4 hours

Ingredients
- 2 tablespoons chili powder
- ½ teaspoon garlic powder
- 1-pound tilapia
- 2 tablespoons lemon juice
- 2 tablespoons olive oil

Instructions
1. Place all ingredients in a mixing bowl. Stir to combine everything.
2. Allow to marinate in the fridge for at least 30 minutes.
3. Get a foil and place the fish including the marinade in the middle of the foil.
4. Fold the foil and crimp the edges to seal.
5. Place inside the crockpot.
6. Cook on high for 2 hours or on low for 4 hours.

Nutrition information: Calories per serving: 183; Carbohydrates: 2.9g; Protein: 23.4g; Fat: 11.3g; Sugar: 0.3g; Sodium: 215mg; Fiber:1.4 g

Spicy Curried Shrimps

Serves: 4
Preparation time: 3 minutes
Cooking time: 2 hours

Ingredients
- 1 ½ pounds shrimp, shelled and deveined
- 1 tablespoon ghee or butter, melted
- 1 tablespoon curry powder
- 1 teaspoon cayenne pepper
- Salt and pepper to taste

Instructions
1. Place all ingredients in the crockpot.
2. Give a stir to incorporate everything.
3. Close the lid and allow to cook on low for 2 hours or on high for 30 minutes.

Nutrition information: Calories per serving: 207; Carbohydrates:2.2 g; Protein: 35.2g; Fat: 10.5g; Sugar: 0g; Sodium: 325mg; Fiber: 1.6g

Crockpot Smoked Trout

Serves: 4
Preparation time: 3 minutes
Cooking time: 2 hours

Ingredients
- 2 tablespoons liquid smoke
- 2 tablespoons olive oil
- 4 ounces smoked trout, skin removed then flaked
- Salt and pepper to taste
- 2 tablespoons mustard

Instructions
1. Place all ingredients in the crockpot.
2. Cook on high for 1 hour or on low for 2 hours until the trout flakes have absorbed the sauce.

Nutrition information: Calories per serving: 116; Carbohydrates: 1.5g; Protein: 7.2g; Fat: 9.2g; Sugar: 0g; Sodium: 347mg; Fiber: 1.3g

Thyme and Sesame Halibut

Serves: 2
Preparation time: 2 hours 5 minutes
Cooking time: 4 hours

Ingredients
- 1 tablespoon lemon juice
- 1 teaspoon thyme
- Salt and pepper to taste
- 8 ounces halibut or mahi-mahi, cut into 2 portions
- 1 tablespoons sesame seeds, toasted

Instructions
1. Line the bottom of the crockpot with a foil.
2. Mix lemon juice, thyme, salt and pepper in a shallow dish.
3. Place the fish and allow to marinate for 2 hours in the fish.
4. Sprinkle the fish with toasted sesame seeds.
5. Arrange the fish in the foil-lined crockpot.
6. Close the lid and cook on high for 2 hours or on low for 4 hours.

Nutrition information: Calories per serving: 238; Carbohydrates: 3.9g; Protein: 23.1g; Fat: 14.9g; Sugar: 0.5g; Sodium:313 mg; Fiber:1.6 g

Salmon with Green Peppercorn Sauce

Serves: 4
Preparation time: 5 minutes
Cooking time: 3 hours

Ingredients
- 1 ¼ pounds salmon fillets, skin removed and cut into 4 portions
- Salt and pepper to taste
- 4 teaspoons unsalted butter
- ¼ cup lemon juice
- 1 teaspoon green peppercorns in vinegar

Instructions
1. Sprinkle the salmon fillets with salt and pepper to taste.
2. In a skillet, heat the butter and sear the salmon fillets for 2 minutes on each side.
3. Transfer in the crockpot and pour the lemon juice and green peppercorns.
4. Adjust the seasoning by adding in more salt or pepper depending on your taste.
5. Close the lid and cook on high for 1 hour or on low for 3 hours.

Nutrition information: Calories per serving: 255; Carbohydrates: 2.3g; Protein: 37.4g; Fat: 13.5g; Sugar: 0g; Sodium: 352mg; Fiber: 1.5g

Coconut Curry Cod

Serves: 4
Preparation time: 3 minutes
Cooking time: 4 hours

Ingredients
- 4 pieces of cod fillets
- Salt and pepper to taste
- 1 ½ cups coconut milk
- 2 teaspoons curry paste
- 2 teaspoons grated ginger

Instructions
1. Place all ingredients in the crockpot.
2. Give a good stir.
3. Close the lid and cook on high for 2 hours or on low for 4 hours.
4. Garnish with chopped cilantro if desired.

Nutrition information: Calories per serving: 296; Carbohydrates: 6.7g; Protein: 20.1g; Fat: 22.8g; Sugar: 2.3g; Sodium:357 mg; Fiber: 3.8g

Almond-Crusted Tilapia

Serves: 4
Preparation time: 5 minutes
Cooking time: 4 hours

Ingredients
- 2 tablespoons olive oil
- 1 cup chopped almonds
- ¼ cup ground flaxseed
- 4 tilapia fillets
- Salt and pepper to taste

Instructions
1. Line the bottom of the crockpot with a foil.
2. Grease the foil with the olive oil.
3. In a mixing bowl, combine the almonds and flaxseed.
4. Season the tilapia with salt and pepper to taste.
5. Dredge the tilapia fillets with the almond and flaxseed mixture.
6. Place neatly in the foil-lined crockpot.
7. Close the lid and cook on high for 2 hours and on low for 4 hours.

Nutrition information: Calories per serving: 233; Carbohydrates: 4.6g; Protein: 25.5g; Fat: 13.3g; Sugar: 0.4g; Sodium: 342mg; Fiber: 1.9g

Buttered Bacon and Scallops

Serves: 4
Preparation time: 5 minutes
Cooking time: 2 hours

Ingredients
- 1 tablespoon butter
- 2 cloves of garlic, chopped
- 24 scallops, rinsed and patted dry
- Salt and pepper to taste
- 1 cup bacon, chopped

Instructions
1. In a skillet, heat the butter and sauté the garlic until fragrant and lightly browned.
2. Transfer to a crockpot and add the scallops.
3. Season with salt and pepper to taste.
4. Close the lid and cook on high for 45 minutes or on low for 2 hours.
5. Meanwhile, cook the bacon until the fat has rendered and crispy.
6. Sprinkle the cooked scallops with crispy bacon.

Nutrition information: Calories per serving: 261; Carbohydrates:4.9 g; Protein:24.7 g; Fat:14.3 g; Sugar: 1.3g; Sodium: 425mg; Fiber: 3g

Lemony Shrimps in Hoisin Sauce

Serves: 4
Preparation time: 3 minutes
Cooking time: 2 hours

Ingredients

- 1/3 cup hoisin sauce
- ½ cup lemon juice, freshly squeezed
- 1 ½ pounds shrimps, shelled and deveined
- Salt and pepper to taste
- 2 tablespoon cilantro leaves, chopped

Instructions

1. Into the crockpot, place the hoisin sauce, lemon juice, and shrimps.
2. Season with salt and pepper to taste.
3. Mix to incorporate all ingredients.
4. Close the lid and cook on high for 30 minutes or on low for 2 hours.
5. Garnish with cilantro leaves.

Nutrition information: Calories per serving: 228; Carbohydrates: 6.3g; Protein: 35.8g; Fat: 3.2g; Sugar: 0g; Sodium: 482mg; Fiber: 4.8g

Bacon-Wrapped Shrimps

Serves: 4
Preparation time: 5 minutes
Cooking time: 2 hours

Ingredients

- 2 tablespoons butter, melted
- 30 large shrimps, shelled
- ½ teaspoon garlic powder
- Salt and pepper to taste
- 15 strips bacon, cut lengthwise

Instructions

1. Line the crockpot bottom with foil.
2. Pour the butter into the crockpot.
3. Marinate the shrimps with garlic powder, salt and pepper. Allow to stay in the fridge for 30 minutes.
4. Wrap the shrimps with bacon and arrange in the crockpot.
5. Close the lid and cook on low for 2 hours or on high for 45 minutes.
6. Be sure to flip the shrimps to sear the other side.

Nutrition information: Calories per serving: 152; Carbohydrates: 3.2g; Protein: 9.5g; Fat: 11.9g; Sugar: 0.5g; Sodium: 492mg; Fiber: 1.7g

Spicy Cajun Scallops

Serves: 6
Preparation time: 3 minutes
Cooking time: 2 hours

Ingredients

- 2 pounds scallops
- 2 teaspoon Cajun seasoning
- 2 tablespoons unsalted butter
- 1 teaspoon cayenne pepper
- Salt and pepper to taste

Instructions

1. Place everything in the crockpot.
2. Give a stir to combine all ingredients.
3. Close the lid and cook on low for 2 hours or on high for 45 minutes.

Nutrition information: Calories per serving: 135; Carbohydrates: 2g; Protein: 19.5g; Fat: 7.2g; Sugar: 0g; Sodium: 384mg; Fiber: 1.4g

Crockpot Greek Snapper

Serves: 8
Preparation time: 5 minutes
Cooking time: 4 hours

Ingredients

- 3 tablespoons olive oil
- 12 snapper fillets
- 1 tablespoon Greek seasoning
- 24 lemon slices
- Salt and pepper to taste

Instructions

1. Line the bottom of the crockpot with foil.
2. Grease the foil with olive oil
3. Season the snapper fillets with Greek seasoning, salt, and pepper.
4. Arrange lemon slices on top.
5. Close the lid and cook on high for 2 hours and on low for 4 hours.

Nutrition information: Calories per serving: 409; Carbohydrates: 4.3g; Protein:67 g; Fat: 15.3g; Sugar: 0g; Sodium: 246mg; Fiber: 1.8g

Shrimps in Coconut Milk

Serves: 4
Cook Time: 3 hours

Ingredients

- 1-pound shrimps, shelled and deveined
- 1 tablespoon minced garlic
- 1 tablespoon grated ginger
- ½ teaspoon turmeric powder
- 1 teaspoon garam masala
- ½ teaspoon cayenne pepper
- ½ can coconut milk, unsweetened
- Salt and pepper to taste

Instructions

1. Place all ingredients in the CrockPot.
2. Give a good stir.
3. Close the lid and cook on high for 2 hours or on low for 3 hours.

Nutrition information: Calories per serving: 192; Carbohydrates: 2g; Protein: 16g; Fat: 12g; Sugar: 0g; Sodium: 481mg; Fiber: 1.3g

Basil-Parmesan Shrimps

Serves: 4
Cook Time: 3 hours

Ingredients

- 1 tablespoon grass-fed butter, melted
- 1-pound shrimps, shelled and deveined
- 2 cloves of garlic, minced
- 2 tablespoons lemon juice, freshly squeezed
- 1 cup grass-fed heavy cream
- ½ cup fresh basil leaves, chopped
- Salt and pepper to taste
- 1 cup organic parmesan cheese, grated

Instructions

1. Place butter in the CrockPot. Add in the shrimps, garlic, and lemon juice on top. Mix until combined.
2. Stir in the cream and basil leaves. Season with salt and pepper to taste.
3. Sprinkle parmesan cheese on top.
4. Close the lid and cook on high for 2 hours or on low for 3 hours.

Nutrition information: Calories per serving:428; Carbohydrates: 3g; Protein: 29g; Fat: 33g; Sugar: 0.4g; Sodium: 510mg; Fiber: 0.8g

Creamy Garlic Shrimps with Goat Cheese

Serves: 4
Cook Time: 3 hours

Ingredients

- 1-pound shrimps, shelled and deveined
- 2 tablespoons butter
- 4 cloves of garlic, minced
- 1 teaspoon paprika
- 1 onion, minced
- ¼ teaspoon cayenne pepper
- 1 teaspoon lemon juice
- Salt and pepper to taste
- ¼ cup organic goat cheese

Instructions

1. Place all ingredients in the CrockPot.
2. Give a good stir.
3. Close the lid and cook on high for 2 hours or on low for 3 hours.

Nutrition information: Calories per serving: 512; Carbohydrates: 3.6g; Protein: 59.2g; Fat: 26.8g; Sugar: 1.2g; Sodium: 891mg; Fiber: 1g

CrockPot Crab Chowder

Serves: 4
Cook Time: 3 hours

Ingredients

- 1 tablespoon butter
- 4 ounces cauliflower stalks, diced
- 1 onion, diced
- 1 stalk of celery, diced
- 1 clove of garlic, crushed
- ¼ teaspoon dried thyme
- 1/8 teaspoon crushed red pepper flakes
- 8 ounces clam juice
- 1 ½ cup heavy cream
- 1 cup almond milk
- 8 ounces crab meat, cooked and shells removed
- Salt and pepper to taste
- 2 tablespoons fresh chives, chopped

Instructions

1. Place all ingredients except for the chives in the CrockPot.
2. Give a good stir.
3. Close the lid and cook on high for 2 hours or on low for 3 hours.
4. Garnish with chives.

Nutrition information: Calories per serving: 480; Carbohydrates: 4g; Protein: 13.6g; Fat: 4.7g; Sugar: 0g; Sodium: 904mg; Fiber: 1g

Red Thai Salmon Curry

Serves: 4
Cook Time: 4 hours

Ingredients

- 2 onions, chopped
- 4 salmon fillets
- 1 can coconut milk
- 1 teaspoon coconut oil
- 1 tablespoon curry powder
- 3 curry leaves
- 1 teaspoon coriander powder
- 1 teaspoon cayenne pepper
- ½ teaspoon cumin
- 1 teaspoon cinnamon
- 2 red bell peppers, julienned

Instructions

1. Place all ingredients in the CrockPot.
2. Give a good stir.
3. Close the lid and cook on high for 3 hours or on low for 4 hours.

Nutrition information: Calories per serving: 499; Carbohydrates: 5.7g; Protein: 27.6g; Fat: 38.3g; Sugar: 0.8g; Sodium: 891mg; Fiber: 3.2g

Prawns in Spicy Coconut Sauce

Serves: 2
Cook Time: 3 hours

Ingredients

- 15 large prawns, peeled
- 2 tablespoons coconut oil
- 1 teaspoon chili powder
- 1 tablespoon lime juice
- ¼ cup cilantro leaves, chopped
- ½ cup coconut milk
- 1 tomato
- ½-inch ginger root, grated
- 4 cloves of garlic, minced

Instructions

1. Place all ingredients in the CrockPot.
2. Give a good stir.
3. Close the lid and cook on high for 2 hours or on low for 3 hours.

Nutrition information: Calories per serving: 673; Carbohydrates: 2.5g; Protein:24.3g; Fat: 63g; Sugar: 0g; Sodium: 810mg; Fiber:0.5g

CrockPot Shrimp Gambas

Serves: 4
Cook Time: 3 hours

Ingredients

- 1/3 cup extra virgin olive oil
- 5 cloves of garlic, chopped
- 1 teaspoon red pepper flakes
- 1 ¼ pounds shrimps, peeled and deveined
- 1 ¼ teaspoon Spanish paprika
- Salt and pepper to taste
- 2 tablespoons parsley, chopped

Instructions

1. Place all ingredients in the CrockPot.
2. Give a good stir.
3. Close the lid and cook on high for 2 hours or on low for 3 hours.

Nutrition information: Calories per serving: 228; Carbohydrates: 3.8g; Protein: 29.8g; Fat: 12.6g; Sugar: 0g; Sodium: 633mg; Fiber: 2.1g

Thai Coconut Shrimps

Serves: 2
Cook Time: 3 hours

Ingredients

- 1 ½ cups coconut milk
- 3 kaffir lime leaves
- 1 lemon grass stalk
- 1 cup fresh cilantro
- 1-inch ginger or galangal root
- 1-pound shrimps, shelled and deveined
- 1 tablespoon coconut oil
- 1 cup mushrooms, sliced
- 1 onion, sliced
- 1 tablespoon fish sauce
- Juice from 1 lime

Instructions

1. Place all ingredients in the CrockPot.
2. Give a good stir.
3. Close the lid and cook on high for 2 hours or on low for 3 hours.
4. Garnish with cilantro.

Nutrition information: Calories per serving: 493; Carbohydrates: 4g; Protein: 11.5g; Fat: 45.3g; Sugar:0 g; Sodium: 940mg; Fiber: 1.7g

Scallops in Lemon Butter Sauce

Serves: 4
Cook Time: 3 hours

Ingredients

- 1-pound scallops, cleaned and patted dry
- Salt and pepper to taste
- 2 tablespoons olive oil
- 4 tablespoons butter
- 3 tablespoons lemon juice, freshly squeezed
- ¼ cup parsley, chopped

Instructions

1. Place all ingredients in the CrockPot.
2. Give a good stir.
3. Close the lid and cook on high for 2 hours or on low for 3 hours.
4. Garnish with parsley.

Nutrition information: Calories per serving: 248; Carbohydrates: 2.1g; Protein: 14.7g; Fat: 18.9g; Sugar: 0g; Sodium: 791mg; Fiber: 0.6g

Tuna Spinach Casserole

Serves: 5
Cook Time: 6 hours

Ingredients

- 1-pound tuna, chopped or ground finely
- 1-inch ginger grated
- 1 tablespoon lemon juice
- 2 tablespoons soy sauce
- Zest from ½ lemon
- ¼ cup butter, melted
- 4 cloves of garlic, minced
- 1 cup heavy cream
- 9 ounces spinach, rinsed and drained
- 4 eggs, beaten
- Salt and pepper to taste
- 1 cup mozzarella cheese

Instructions

1. In a mixing bowl, combine the tuna, ginger, lemon juice, soy sauce, and lemon zest. Marinate for at least 2 hours in the fridge.
2. After 2 hours, discard the juices of the tuna and transfer into the CrockPot.
3. Stir in the butter, garlic, heavy cream, and spinach. Add in the beaten eggs and season with salt and pepper to taste.
4. Sprinkle mozzarella cheese on top.
5. Close the lid and cook on high for 4 hours or on low for 6 hours.

Nutrition information: Calories per serving: 573; Carbohydrates: 2.1g; Protein: 39.1g; Fat:45.3g; Sugar: 0g; Sodium: 761mg; Fiber: 1.2g

Simple CrockPot Steamed Crab

Serves: 2
Cook Time: 3 hours

Ingredients

- 2 pounds medium-sized crabs, cleaned
- Juice from 1 lemon, freshly squeezed
- ¼ cup water
- 3 tablespoons butter
- 4 cloves of garlic, minced
- 2 onions, chopped
- 2 bay leaves
- Salt and pepper to taste

Instructions

1. Place all ingredients in the CrockPot.
2. Give a good stir.
3. Close the lid and cook on high for 2 hours or on low for 3 hours.

Nutrition information: Calories per serving: 392; Carbohydrates: 2.1g; Protein: 38.2g; Fat: 27.5g; Sugar: 0g; Sodium: 819mg; Fiber: 1.6g

CrockPot Seafood Jambalaya

Serves: 7
Cook Time: 3 hours

Ingredients

- 1 onion, chopped
- 2 tablespoons olive oil
- 2 ribs of celery, sliced
- 1 green bell pepper, seeded and chopped
- 1 cup tomatoes, crushed
- 1 cup chicken broth
- 2 teaspoons dried oregano
- 2 teaspoons dried parsley
- 2 teaspoons organic Cajun seasoning
- 1 teaspoon cayenne pepper
- 1-pound shrimps, shelled and deveined
- ½ pound squid, cleaned
- 2 cups grated cauliflower

Instructions

1. Place all ingredients in the CrockPot.
2. Give a good stir.
3. Close the lid and cook on high for 2 hours or on low for 3 hours.

Nutrition information: Calories per serving: 205; Carbohydrates: 5.9g; Protein: 26.7g; Fat: 10.5g; Sugar: 0.2g; Sodium: 830mg; Fiber: 3.2g

CrockPot Fish Chowder

Serves: 9
Cook Time: 3 hours

Ingredients

- 2 pounds catfish fillet, sliced
- 2 tablespoons butter
- ½ cup fresh oysters
- 1 onion, chopped
- 2 cups water
- 1 red bell pepper, chopped
- 1 yellow bell pepper, chopped
- Salt and pepper to taste
- 1 cup full-fat milk

Instructions

1. Place all ingredients in the CrockPot.
2. Give a good stir.
3. Close the lid and cook on high for 2 hours or on low for 3 hours.

Nutrition information: Calories per serving: 172; Carbohydrates:6.1 g; Protein: 20.5g; Fat: 9.4g; Sugar: 1.3g; Sodium: 592mg; Fiber: 3.5g

CrockPot Seafood Cioppino

Serves: 8
Cook Time: 4 hours

Ingredients

- 1-pound haddock fillets, cut into strips
- 1-pound shrimps, shelled and deveined
- 1 cup raw clam meat
- 1 cup crab meat
- 1 cup tomatoes, diced
- 2 onions, chopped
- 3 stalks of celery, chopped
- 2 cups clam juice
- 3 tablespoons tomato paste
- 5 cloves of garlic, minced
- 1 tablespoons olive oil
- 2 teaspoons Italian seasoning
- 1 bay leaf

Instructions

1. Place all ingredients in the CrockPot.
2. Give a good stir.
3. Close the lid and cook on high for 3 hours or on low for 4 hours.
4. Garnish with parsley.

Nutrition information: Calories per serving: 217; Carbohydrates: 5.2g; Protein: 26.8g; Fat: 8.1g; Sugar: 0g; Sodium: 620mg; Fiber: 3.5g

CrockPot Manhattan-Style Clam Chowder

Serves: 4
Cook Time: 3 hours

Ingredients

- 1 cup onion, chopped
- 2 cups nitrate-free bacon
- 3 ribs of celery, chopped
- 1 tablespoon parsley, chopped
- 1 ½ cups tomatoes, crushed
- 1 bay leaf
- 1 teaspoon dried thyme
- 2 cups diced clams, drained
- 1 can clam juice
- 1 tablespoon melted butter
- Salt and pepper to taste

Instructions

1. Place all ingredients in the CrockPot.
2. Give a good stir.
3. Close the lid and cook on high for 2 hours or on low for 3 hours.
4. Garnish with chopped parsley if desired.

Nutrition information: Calories per serving: 365; Carbohydrates: 6.3g; Protein: 34.1g; Fat: 28.4g; Sugar: 0.5g; Sodium: 728mg; Fiber: 4.3g

CrockPot Tuna Spaghetti

Serves: 3
Cook Time: 2 hours

Ingredients

- 2 stalks of celery, chopped
- 1/3 cup chicken broth
- 1 cup full-fat milk
- 2 tablespoons parsley flakes
- ½ pound ground tuna, boiled
- 2 zucchinis, spiralized or cut into long strips
- 1 tablespoons butter
- Salt and pepper to taste

Instructions

1. Place all ingredients in the CrockPot.
2. Give a good stir.
3. Close the lid and cook on high for 1 hours or on low for 2 hours.
4. Garnish with chopped parsley if desired.

Nutrition information: Calories per serving: 320; Carbohydrates:7.3 g; Protein: 30.9g; Fat: 19.3g; Sugar: 0.2g; Sodium: 590mg; Fiber: 4.8g

CrockPot Garlic Shrimps

Serves: 5
Cook Time: 3 hours

Ingredients

- 4 tablespoons butter
- ¼ cup olive oil
- 5 cloves of garlic, minced
- ½ teaspoon salt
- ¼ teaspoon black pepper
- 1 ½ pounds jumbo shrimps, shelled and deveined.

Instructions

1. Place all ingredients in the CrockPot.
2. Give a good stir.
3. Close the lid and cook on high for 2 hours or on low for 3 hours.
4. Garnish with chopped parsley if desired.

Nutrition information: Calories per serving: 292; Carbohydrates: 1.1g; Protein:27.6 g; Fat: 20.7g; Sugar: 0g; Sodium: 401mg; Fiber: 0.6g

CrockPot Creole Seafood

Serves: 6
Cook Time: 3 hours

Ingredients

- 3 tablespoons olive oil
- 2 cloves of garlic, minced
- 2 stalks of celery, chopped
- 1 ½ cups tomatoes, crushed
- 1 bay leaf
- 1 teaspoon thyme
- A dash of Tabasco sauce
- ½ pound catfish fillets, cut into strips
- ½ pound shrimps, shelled and deveined
- Salt and pepper to taste

Instructions

1. Place all ingredients in the CrockPot.
2. Give a good stir.
3. Close the lid and cook on high for 2 hours or on low for 3 hours.
4. Garnish with chopped green onions if desired.

Nutrition information: Calories per serving: 146; Carbohydrates: 2.6g; Protein:15.4g; Fat: 8.4g; Sugar: 0g; Sodium: 419mg; Fiber: 1.6g

CrockPot Asian Shrimps

Serves: 2
Cook Time: 3 hours
Ingredients
- ½ cup chicken stock
- 2 tablespoons soy sauce
- ½ teaspoon sliced ginger
- ½ pound shrimps, cleaned and deveined
- 2 tablespoons rice vinegar
- 2 tablespoons sesame oil
- 2 tablespoons toasted sesame seeds
- 2 tablespoons green onions, chopped

Instructions
1. Place the chicken stock, soy sauce, ginger, shrimps, and rice vinegar in the CrockPot.
2. Give a good stir.
3. Close the lid and cook on high for 2 hours or on low for 3 hours.
4. Sprinkle with sesame oil, sesame seeds, and chopped green onions before serving.

Nutrition information: Calories per serving: 352; Carbohydrates: 4.7g; Protein: 30.2g; Fat: 24.3g; Sugar: 0.4g; Sodium: 755mg; Fiber: 2.9g

CrockPot Fish and Tomatoes

Serves: 2
Cook Time: 5 hours
Ingredients
- 1-pound cod fillets, cut into large chunks
- 1 bell pepper, sliced
- 3 cloves of garlic, minced
- 1 onion, chopped
- 3 tablespoons butter
- 1 cup tomatoes, crushed
- 1 tablespoon rosemary
- ¼ cup chicken broth
- ¼ teaspoon red pepper flakes
- Salt and pepper to taste.

Instructions
1. Place the ingredients in the CrockPot.
2. Give a good stir.
3. Close the lid and cook on high for 4 hours or on low for 5 hours.
4. Sprinkle with sesame oil, sesame seeds, and chopped green onions before serving.

Nutrition information: Calories per serving:420; Carbohydrates: 7.3g; Protein: 43.9g; Fat: 25.6g; Sugar: 0g; Sodium: 932mg; Fiber: 3.4g

Crockpot Chicken Curry

Serves: 6
Preparation time: 3 minutes
Cooking time: 8 hours

Ingredients

- 2 pounds chicken breasts, bones removed
- 1 can coconut milk
- 1 onion, chopped
- 4 tablespoons curry powder
- Salt and pepper to taste

Instructions

1. Place all ingredients in the crockpot.
2. Give a good stir to incorporate everything.
3. Close the lid and cook on low for 8 hours or 6 hours on high.

Nutrition information: Calories per serving:468; Carbohydrates: 9g; Protein: 34.5g; Fat: 33.7g; Sugar: 1.2g; Sodium:646 mg; Fiber: 1.6g

Cheesy Ranch Chicken

Serves: 6
Preparation time: 5 minutes
Cooking time: 8 hours

Ingredients

- 1 ¼ pounds chicken breasts, bones removed
- ½ cup sugar-free ranch dressing
- ½ cup cheddar cheese, shredded
- ½ cup parmesan cheese, shredded
- Cayenne pepper to taste

Instructions

1. Pour the ranch dressing in the crockpot.
2. Arrange the chicken pieces on top.
3. Sprinkle a dash of cayenne pepper to taste.
4. Add the two cheeses on top.
5. Close the lid and cook on low for 8 hours or on high for 6 hours.

Nutrition information: Calories per serving: 267; Carbohydrates: 7g; Protein: 25g; Fat: 15.1g; Sugar: 2.4g; Sodium:673 mg; Fiber: 1.7g

Lemon Parsley Chicken

Serves: 4
Preparation time: 5 minutes
Cooking time: 8 hours

Ingredients

- 2 tablespoons butter, melted
- 1-pound chicken breasts, bones removed
- Salt and pepper to taste
- 1 lemon, sliced thinly
- ½ cup parsley, chopped

Instructions

1. Line the bottom of the crockpot with foil.
2. Grease the foil with melted butter.
3. Season the chicken breasts with salt and pepper to taste.
4. Arrange on the foil and place lemon slices on top.
5. Sprinkle with chopped parsley.
6. Cook on low for 8 hours or on high for 6 hours

Nutrition information: Calories per serving: 303; Carbohydrates: 3.1g; Protein: 34.5g; Fat: 14g; Sugar: 0.7g; Sodium: 430mg; Fiber: 1g

Lemon Garlic Dump Chicken

Serves: 6
Preparation time: 9 minutes
Cooking time: 8 hours

Ingredients

- ¼ cup olive oil
- 2 teaspoon garlic, minced
- 6 chicken breasts, bones removed
- 1 tablespoon parsley, chopped
- 2 tablespoons lemon juice, freshly squeezed

Instructions

1. Heat oil in a skillet over medium flame.
2. Sauté the garlic until golden brown.
3. Arrange the chicken breasts in the crockpot.
4. Pour over the oil with garlic.
5. Add the parsley and lemon juice. Add a little water.
6. Close the lid and cook on low for 8 hours or on high for 6 hours.

Nutrition information: Calories per serving: 581; Carbohydrates: 0.7g; Protein: 60.5g; Fat: 35.8g; Sugar: 0g; Sodium: 583mg; Fiber: 0.3g

Harissa Chicken Breasts

Serves: 6
Preparation time: 3 minutes
Cooking time: 8 hours

Ingredients
- 1 tablespoon olive oil
- 1-pound chicken breasts, skin and bones removed
- Salt to taste
- 2 tablespoon Harissa or Sriracha sauce
- 2 tablespoons toasted sesame seeds

Instructions
1. Pour oil in the crockpot.
2. Arrange the chicken breasts and season with salt and pepper to taste
3. Stir in the Sriracha or Harissa sauce. Give a good stir to incorporate everything.
4. Close the lid and cook on low for 8 hours or on high for 6 hours.
5. Once cooked, sprinkle toasted sesame seeds on top.

Nutrition information: Calories per serving: 167; Carbohydrates: 1.1g; Protein: 16.3g; Fat: 10.6g; Sugar: 0g; Sodium: 632mg; Fiber: 0.6g

Cilantro Lime Chicken

Serves: 3
Preparation time: 3 minutes
Cooking time: 8 hours

Ingredients
- 3 chicken breasts, bones and skin removed
- Juice from 3 limes, freshly squeezed
- 6 cloves of garlic, minced
- 1 teaspoon cumin
- ¼ cup cilantro

Instructions
1. Place all ingredients in the crockpot.
2. Give a stir to mix everything.
3. Close the lid and cook on low for 8 hours or on high for 6 hours.

Nutrition information: Calories per serving: 522; Carbohydrates: 6.1g; Protein: 61.8g; Fat: 27.1g; Sugar: 2.3g; Sodium: 453mg; Fiber: 1.2g

Asian Sesame Chicken

Serves: 12
Preparation time: 3 minutes
Cooking time: 8 hours

Ingredients
- 12 chicken thighs, bones and skin removed
- 2 tablespoons sesame oil
- 3 tablespoons water
- 3 tablespoons soy sauce
- 1 thumb-size ginger, sliced thinly

Instructions
1. Place all ingredients in the crockpot.
2. Stir all ingredients to combine.
3. Close the lid and cook on low for 8 hours or on high for 6 hours.
4. Once cooked, garnish with toasted sesame seeds.

Nutrition information: Calories per serving: 458; Carbohydrates: 1.5g; Protein: 32.2g; Fat: 35.05g; Sugar: 0g; Sodium: 426mg; Fiber: 0.4g

Turkey with Zucchini

Serves: 4
Preparation time: 3 minutes
Cooking time: 8 hours

Ingredients
- 1-pound ground turkey
- 2 red peppers cut into strips
- Salt and pepper to taste
- 2 green onions, sliced
- 1 large zucchini, sliced

Instructions
1. Place the ground turkey and red peppers in the crockpot.
2. Season with salt and pepper to taste.
3. Close the lid and cook on low for 8 hours or on high for 6 hours.
4. An hour before the cooking time is done, stir in the green onions and zucchini.
5. Cook further until the vegetables are soft.

Nutrition information: Calories per serving: 195; Carbohydrates: 5.7g; Protein: 23.9g; Fat: 9.01g; Sugar: 0.4g; Sodium: 542mg; Fiber: 2.5g

Chicken, Peppers and Onions

Serves: 4
Preparation time: 8 minutes
Cooking time: 8 hours

Ingredients

- 1 tablespoon olive oil
- ½ cup shallots, peeled
- 1-pound boneless chicken breasts, sliced
- ½ cup green and red peppers, diced
- Salt and pepper to taste

Instructions

1. Heat oil in a skillet over medium flame.
2. Sauté the shallots until fragrant and translucent. Allow to cook so that the outer edges of the shallots turn slightly brown. Transfer into the crockpot.
3. Add the chicken breasts and the peppers.
4. Season with salt and pepper to taste. Add a few tablespoons of water.
5. Close the lid and cook on low for 8 hours or on high for 6 hours.

Nutrition information: Calories per serving: 179; Carbohydrates: 3.05g; Protein:26.1 g; Fat: 10.4g; Sugar: 0g; Sodium: 538mg; Fiber:2.4 g

Almond-Stuffed Chicken

Serves: 6
Preparation time: 10 minutes
Cooking time: 8 hours

Ingredients

- 1 ½ teaspoons butter
- 1/3 cup Boursin cheese or any herbed cheese of your choice
- ¼ cup slivered almonds, toasted and chopped
- 4 boneless chicken breasts, halved
- Salt and pepper to taste

Instructions

1. Line the bottom of the crockpot with foil. Grease the foil with butter.
2. In a mixing bowl, mix together the cheese and almonds.
3. Cut a slit through the chicken breasts to create a pocket.
4. Season the chicken with salt and pepper to taste.
5. Spoon the cheese mixture into the slit on the chicken. Secure the slit with toothpicks. Place the chicken in the foil-lined crockpot.
6. Cover with lid and cook on low for 8 hours or on high for 6 hours.

Nutrition information: Calories per serving: 249; Carbohydrates: 0.9g; Protein: 42.1g; Fat: 10g; Sugar: 0g; Sodium:592 mg; Fiber:0.4 g

Rosemary Rotisserie Chicken

Serves: 12
Preparation time: 12 hours
Cooking time: 12 hours

Ingredients
- 1-gallon water
- ¾ cup salt
- ½ cup butter
- 2 tablespoons rosemary and other herbs of your choice
- 1 whole chicken, excess fat removed

Instructions
1. In a pot, combine the water, salt, sugar, and herbs.
2. Stir to dissolve the salt and sugar.
3. Submerge the chicken completely and allow to sit in the brine for 12 hours inside the fridge.
4. Line the crockpot with tin foil.
5. Place the chicken and cook on low for 12 hours or on high for 7 hours.

Nutrition information: Calories per serving: 194; Carbohydrates: 1.4g; Protein:20.6 g; Fat:6.2g; Sugar: 0g; Sodium: 562mg; Fiber: 0.9g

Simple Buttered Rosemary Chicken Breasts

Serves: 4
Preparation time: 8 minutes
Cooking time: 6 hours
Ingredients
- 5 tablespoons butter
- 4 boneless chicken breasts
- Salt and pepper to taste
- 1 tablespoon parsley
- 1 teaspoon rosemary

Instructions
1. Melt the butter in the skillet.
2. Season chicken with salt and pepper to taste. Brown all sides of the chicken for 3 minutes.
3. Transfer into the crockpot and sprinkle with parsley and rosemary.
4. Cook on low for 6 hours or on high for 5 hours.

Nutrition information: Calories per serving: 459; Carbohydrates: 1.17g; Protein: 61.6g; Fat: 21.5g; Sugar: 0g; Sodium: 527mg; Fiber: 0.6g

Curry-Glazed Chicken

Serves: 12
Preparation time: 3 minutes
Cooking time: 9 hours

Ingredients
- ¼ cup butter, melted
- ¼ cup yellow mustard
- Salt and pepper to taste
- 2 tablespoons curry powder
- 1 whole chicken, cut up into pieces

Instructions
1. Place all ingredients in the crockpot.
2. Mix everything to combine.
3. Close the lid and cook on low for 9 hours or on high for 7 hours.

Nutrition information: Calories per serving: 119; Carbohydrates:3.5 g; Protein: 10.5g; Fat: 8.5g; Sugar: 0g; Sodium: 325mg; Fiber: 1.6g

Crockpot Roasted Chicken

Serves: 8
Preparation time: 5 minutes
Cooking time: 8 hours

Ingredients
- 2 tablespoons olive oil
- 8 chicken breasts, skin and bones removed
- 1 cup parsley leaves, chopped
- 5 cloves of garlic, sliced
- Salt and pepper to taste

Instructions
1. Place foil in the bottom of the crockpot.
2. Pour the olive oil.
3. Season the chicken breasts with parsley leaves, garlic, salt and pepper.
4. Place in the crockpot and give a good mix.
5. Close the lid and cook on low for 8 hours and on high for 6 hours.

Nutrition information: Calories per serving: 526; Carbohydrates: 1.6g; Protein: 60.9g; Fat: 30.3g; Sugar: 0g; Sodium: 536mg; Fiber:0.7 g

Sun-Dried Tomato Chicken

Serves: 10
Preparation time: 10 minutes
Cooking time: 8 hours

Ingredients
- 1 tablespoon butter
- 3 cloves of garlic, minced
- 4 pounds whole chicken, cut into pieces
- 1 cup sun-dried tomatoes in vinaigrette
- Salt and pepper to taste

Instructions
- In a skillet, melt the butter and sauté the garlic until lightly browned.
- Add the chicken pieces and cook for 3 minutes until slightly browned.
- Transfer to the crockpot and stir in the sun-dried tomatoes including the vinaigrette.
- Season with salt and pepper to taste.
- Close the lid and cook on low for 8 hours or on high for 6 hours.

Nutrition information: Calories per serving: 397; Carbohydrates:9.4 g; Protein: 30.26g; Fat:14.1 g; Sugar: 0.4g; Sodium: 472mg; Fiber: 5.8g

Lime and Pepper Chicken

Serves: 4
Preparation time: 4 hours
Cooking time: 8 hours

Ingredients
- ½ cup lime juice
- Salt and pepper to taste
- 3 tablespoons sucralose or stevia sweetener
- 4 chicken breasts, bones removed
- 1 tablespoon olive oil

Instructions
1. In a mixing bowl, combine the lime juice, salt, pepper, and sucralose.
2. Marinate the chicken breasts for a few hours in the fridge.
3. Add the oil and give a good mix.
4. Close the lid and cook on low for 8 hours or on high for 6 hours.

Nutrition information: Calories per serving: 573; Carbohydrates: 4.7g; Protein:60.3 g; Fat:30.9 g; Sugar: 0g; Sodium: 492mg; Fiber: 3.2g

Chicken Cordon Bleu

Serves: 4
Preparation time: 10 minutes
Cooking time: 8 hours

Ingredients

- 4 chicken breasts, skin and bones removed
- Salt and pepper to taste
- 4 ounces smoked ham, sliced
- 4 ounces gruyere cheese, sliced
- 1 tablespoon olive oil

Instructions

1. Line the bottom of the crockpot with foil.
2. Create a slit on the chicken and thin out the meat.
3. Season the chicken breasts with salt and pepper.
4. Place smoked ham and cheese in the middle of the chicken breasts.
5. Roll the chicken and secure the edges with toothpick.
6. Brush olive oil on the surface of the chicken.
7. Place in the crockpot and cook on low for 8 hours or on high for 6 hours.
8. Remove the toothpicks before serving.

Nutrition information: Calories per serving: 679; Carbohydrates: 1.4g; Protein: 73.9g; Fat: 40.5g; Sugar: 0g; Sodium: 428mg; Fiber: 0g

Crockpot Cheesy Buttermilk Drumsticks

Serves: 8
Preparation time: 5 minutes
Cooking time: 8 hours

Ingredients

- 2 tablespoons butter, melted
- 8 chicken drumsticks
- Salt and pepper to taste
- ¾ cup buttermilk
- 1/3 cup grated parmesan cheese

Instructions

1. Pour melted butter in the crockpot.
2. Season the chicken drumsticks with salt and pepper to taste.
3. Place in the crockpot and pour the buttermilk.
4. Top with parmesan cheese.
5. Close the lid and cook on low for 8 hours and on high for 6 hours.

Nutrition information: Calories per serving: 264; Carbohydrates:2.3 g; Protein: 25.6g; Fat: 16.8g; Sugar: 0.4g; Sodium: 783mg; Fiber:0 g

Crockpot Chicken, Egg and Tomato Stew

Serves: 4
Preparation time: 3 minutes
Cooking time: 8 hours

Ingredients
- 2 tablespoons butter, melted
- 4 chicken breasts, skin and bones removed
- Salt and pepper to taste
- 4 large eggs, unbeaten
- ½ cup organic tomato sauce

Instructions
1. Pour the melted butter in the crockpot.
2. Arrange the chicken pieces and season with salt and pepper to taste.
3. Pour the tomato sauce.
4. Carefully, crack the eggs into the chicken and tomato sauce.
5. Close the lid and cook on high for 8 hours or on low for 6 hours.

Nutrition information: Calories per serving: 616; Carbohydrates: 3.3g; Protein: 63.8g; Fat: 37.2g; Sugar: 0g; Sodium: 637mg; Fiber: 2.4g

Mexican Chicken in Crockpot

Serves: 4
Preparation time: 3 minutes
Cooking time: 8 hours

Ingredients
- 2 tablespoons butter
- 1 can diced tomatoes, undrained
- 2 cups chicken, cubed
- Salt and pepper to taste
- 1 teaspoon cumin

Instructions
1. Place all ingredients in the crockpot.
2. Mix everything to combine.
3. Close the lid and cook on low for 8 hours or on high for 5 hours.
Nutrition information: Calories per serving: 594; Carbohydrates: 2.9g; Protein: 97.3 g; Fat: 21.7g; Sugar: 0.5g; Sodium: 637mg; Fiber: 0.8g

Chicken Vegetable Curry

Serves: 6
Preparation time: 3 minutes
Cooking time: 8 hours

Ingredients
- 1 tablespoon butter
- 1-pound chicken breasts, bones removed
- 1 package frozen vegetable mix
- 1 cup water
- 2 tablespoons curry powder

Instructions
1. Place all ingredients in the crockpot.
2. Stir to combine everything.
3. Close the lid and cook on low for 8 hours or on high for 6 hours.

Nutrition information: Calories per serving: 273; Carbohydrates: 6.1g; Protein:21 g; Fat: 10g; Sugar: 0.1g; Sodium: 311mg; Fiber: 4g

Chicken Enchilada

Serves: 10
Preparation time: 5 minutes
Cooking time: 8 hours

Ingredients
- 4 ½ cups shredded chicken
- 1 ¼ cup sour cream
- 1 can sugar-free green enchilada sauce
- 4 cups Monterey jack cheese
- ½ cup cilantro, chopped

Instructions
1. Place the shredded chicken in the crockpot.
2. Add in the sour cream and enchilada sauce.
3. Sprinkle with Monterey jack cheese.
4. Close the lid and cook on low for 8 hours or on high for 6 hours.
5. An hour before the cooking time ends, sprinkle with cilantro.

Nutrition information: Calories per serving: 469; Carbohydrates: 5g; Protein: 34g; Fat:29 g; Sugar:2.2 g; Sodium: 977mg; Fiber: 1g

Chicken Piccata

Serves: 4
Preparation time: 3 minutes
Cooking time: 8 hours

Ingredients
- 4 chicken breasts, skin and bones removed
- Salt and pepper to taste
- ¼ cup butter, cubed
- ¼ cup chicken broth
- 1 tablespoon lemon juice

Instructions
1. Place all ingredients in the crockpot.
2. Give a good stir to combine everything.
3. Close the lid and cook on low for 8 hours or on high for 6 hours.

Nutrition information: Calories per serving: 265; Carbohydrates:2.3 g; Protein:24 g; Fat: 14g; Sugar: 0g; Sodium:442 mg; Fiber:0 g

Chicken Provolone

Serves: 4
Preparation time: 5 minutes
Cooking time: 8 hours

Ingredients
- 4 chicken breasts, bones and skin removed
- Salt and pepper to taste
- 8 fresh basil leaves
- 4 slices prosciutto
- 4 slices provolone cheese

Instructions
1. Sprinkle the chicken breasts with salt and pepper to taste.
2. Place in the crockpot and add the basil leaves, and prosciutto on top.
3. Arrange the provolone cheese slices on top.
4. Close the lid and cook on low for 8 hours and on high for 6 hours.

Nutrition information: Calories per serving: 236; Carbohydrates: 1g; Protein: 33g; Fat: 11g; Sugar:0 g; Sodium: 435mg; Fiber:0 g

Chicken with Basil and Tomatoes

Serves: 4
Preparation time: 3 minutes
Cooking time: 8 hours

Ingredients
- ¾ cup balsamic vinegar
- ¼ cup fresh basil leaves
- 4 boneless chicken breasts, bone and skin removed
- 2 tablespoons olive oil
- 8 plum tomatoes, sliced

Instructions
1. Place balsamic vinegar, basil leaves, olive oil and tomatoes in a blender. Season with salt and pepper to taste. Pulse until fine.
2. Arrange the chicken pieces in the crockpot.
3. Pour over the sauce.
4. Close the lid and cook on low for 8 hours or on high for 6 hours.

Nutrition information: Calories per serving: 177; Carbohydrates:4 g; Protein:24 g; Fat: 115g; Sugar: 0g; Sodium: 171mg; Fiber: 3.5g

Crockpot Caesar Chicken

Serves: 4
Preparation time: 10 minutes
Cooking time: 8 hours

Ingredients
- ½ cup cashew nuts, soaked in water overnight
- 2 tablespoon Dijon mustard
- 4 boneless chicken breasts, skin and bones removed
- Salt and pepper to taste
- ¼ cup parmesan cheese, divided

Instructions
1. In a blender, place the cashew nuts and Dijon mustard. Season with salt and pepper to taste. Blend until smooth. Set aside.
2. Season the chicken breasts with salt and pepper to taste.
3. Place in the crockpot and add half of the parmesan cheese.
4. Pour over the sauce and mix until well combined.
5. Sprinkle the remaining parmesan cheese.
6. Close the lid and cook on low for 8 hours or on high for 6 hours.

Nutrition information: Calories per serving: 320; Carbohydrates:4.2 g; Protein: 38g; Fat: 12g; Sugar: 1g; Sodium: 530mg; Fiber: 3g

Spicy Almond-Crusted Chicken Nuggets in The Crockpot

Serves: 6
Preparation time: 6 minutes
Cooking time: 8 hours

Ingredients

- ¼ cup butter, melted
- 1 ½ cups almond meal
- 1 ½ cups grated parmesan cheese
- 1 ½ pounds boneless chicken breasts, cut into strips
- 2 eggs, beaten

Instructions

1. Place foil at the bottom of the crockpot.
2. Combine the almond meal and parmesan cheese.
3. Dip the chicken strips into the eggs and dredge into the parmesan and cheese mixture.
4. Place carefully in the crockpot.
5. Close the lid and cook on low for 8 hours or on high for 6 hours.

Nutrition information: Calories per serving: 371; Carbohydrates: 2.5g; Protein:29 g; Fat: 22g; Sugar: 0.8g; Sodium: 527mg; Fiber: 1.4g

Chicken Florentine

Serves: 4
Preparation time: 3 minutes
Cooking time: 8 hours

Ingredients

- 4 chicken breasts, bones and skin removed
- Salt and pepper to taste
- 2 cups parmesan cheese, divided
- ½ cup heavy cream
- 1 cup baby spinach, rinsed

Instructions

1. Place the chicken in the crockpot. Season with salt and pepper to taste.
2. Stir in half of the parmesan cheese.
3. Close the lid and cook on low for 8 hours or on high for 6 hours.
4. Halfway through the cooking time, pour in the heavy cream.
5. Continue cooking.
6. An hour after the cooking time, add in the baby spinach.
7. Cook until the spinach has wilted.

Nutrition information: Calories per serving: 553; Carbohydrates: 3g; Protein: 48g; Fat: 32g; Sugar:0 g; Sodium: 952mg; Fiber: 2.6g

Simple Chicken and Vegetables

Serves: 4
Preparation time: 3 minutes
Cooking time: 8 hours

Ingredients

- 1-pound chicken breasts, bones and skin removed
- 1 sweet red bell pepper, cut into cubes
- 1 zucchini, sliced
- 1 red onion, cut into wedges
- 2/3 cup sun-dried tomatoes in vinaigrette

Instructions

1. Place all ingredients in the crockpot.
2. Give a good stir.
3. Season with salt and pepper to taste.
4. Close the lid and cook on low for 8 hours or on high for 6 hours.

Nutrition information: Calories per serving: 228; Carbohydrates:4.3 g; Protein: 24g; Fat: 15g; Sugar:0 g; Sodium: 55mg; Fiber: 3.7g

Mediterranean Stuffed Chicken

Serves: 4
Preparation time: 10 minutes
Cooking time: 8 hours

Ingredients

- 4 chicken breasts, bones and skin removed
- Salt and pepper to taste
- 1 cup feta cheese, crumbled
- 1/3 cup sun-dried tomatoes, chopped
- 2 tablespoons olive oil

Instructions

1. Create a slit in the chicken breasts to thin out the meat. Season with salt and pepper to taste
2. In a mixing bowl, combine the feta cheese and sun-dried tomatoes.
3. Spoon the feta cheese mixture into the slit created into the chicken.
4. Close the slit using toothpicks.
5. Brush the chicken with olive oil.
6. Place in the crockpot and cook on high for 6 hours or on low for 8 hours.

Nutrition information: Calories per serving: 332; Carbohydrates: 3g; Protein:40 g; Fat: 17g; Sugar: 0g; Sodium: 621mg; Fiber:2.4 g

Chicken Cooked in Coconut Milk and Lemon Grass

Serves: 10
Cook Time: 8 hours

Ingredients

- 10 chicken drumsticks, skin removed
- 1 stalk lemon grass, trimmed and cut into 5 inches long
- 4 cloves of garlic, chopped
- 1 thumb-size ginger, sliced thinly
- 1 cup coconut milk, unsweetened
- 2 tablespoons fish sauce
- 3 tablespoons soy sauce
- 1 teaspoon five spice powder
- 1 onion, sliced
- Salt and pepper to taste
- ¼ cup scallions, chopped

Instructions

1. Place all ingredients except for the scallions in the CrockPot.
2. Close the lid and cook on low high for 6 hours or on low for 8 hours until the chicken is tender.
3. An hour before the cooking time ends, add in the scallions.

Nutrition information: Calories per serving: 285; Carbohydrates: 4.1g; Protein: 24.8g; Fat: 18.7g; Sugar: 0g; Sodium: 538mg; Fiber: 2.7g

Chicken Stew in A CrockPot

Serves: 4
Cook Time: 5 hours

Ingredients

- 2 cups homemade chicken stock
- 2 celery sticks, diced
- ½ onion, diced
- 4 chicken breasts, cut into small pieces
- 3 cloves of garlic, minced
- 1 sprig of rosemary
- ¼ teaspoon dried thyme
- Salt and pepper to taste
- 1 cup fresh spinach
- ½ cup heavy cream

Instructions

1. Place all ingredients except for the spinach and heavy cream in the CrockPot.
2. Close the lid and cook on high for 4 hours or on low for 5 hours.
3. Halfway through the cooking time, add in the spinach and heavy cream.
4. Continue cooking until the chicken is cooked through.

Nutrition information: Calories per serving: 228; Carbohydrates: 3g; Protein: 23g; Fat: 11g; Sugar: 0g; Sodium: 525mg; Fiber: 1.4g

Roasted Chicken with Lemon-Parsley Butter

Serves: 8
Cook Time: 8 hours

Ingredients
- 1 whole roasting chicken
- ½ teaspoon salt
- ¼ teaspoon black pepper
- 1 cup water
- 1 stick of grass-fed butter
- 2 tablespoons parsley, chopped
- 1 whole lemon, sliced

Instructions
1. Season the chicken with salt and pepper.
2. Place inside the CrockPot and pour in 1 cup of water.
3. Close the lid and cook on high for 6 hours or on low for 8 hours.
4. Meanwhile, heat the butter on a skillet over medium flame. Add in the parsley and cook for a minute.
5. Two hours before the cooking time, pour the butter mixture all over the chicken. Arrange lemon slices on top of the chicken.
6. Close the lid and continue cooking until the chicken is tender and cooked through.

Nutrition information: Calories per serving:455; Carbohydrates: 0.5g; Protein: 46.4g; Fat: 29.1g; Sugar: 0g; Sodium: 1184mg; Fiber: 0g

CrockPot Kalua Chicken

Serves: 4
Cook Time: 8 hours

Ingredients
- 2 pounds chicken thighs, bones and skin removed
- 1 tablespoon salt
- 1 tablespoon liquid smoke
- ¼ cup water

Instructions
1. Place all ingredients in the CrockPot.
2. Close the lid and cook on high for 6 hours or on low for 8 hours.
3. Once cooked, serve with organic sour cream, avocado slices, and cilantro if desired.

Nutrition information: Calories per serving: 501; Carbohydrates: 0.6g; Protein: 37.8g; Fat: 36.4g; Sugar: 0g; Sodium: 930mg; Fiber: 0g

Creamy Mexican CrockPot Chicken

Serves: 6
Cook Time: 8 hours

Ingredients

- 1 cup organic sour cream
- ½ cup chicken stock
- 1 cup tomatoes, diced
- 1 green chili, chopped
- ½ teaspoon cumin
- ½ teaspoon oregano
- ½ teaspoon cayenne pepper
- 2 pounds chicken breasts
- A sprig of cilantro, chopped

Instructions

1. Place all ingredients except for the cilantro in the CrockPot.
2. Close the lid and cook on high for 6 hours or on low for 8 hours.
3. Garnish with cilantro.

Nutrition information: Calories per serving: 262; Carbohydrates: 4.3g; Protein: 32g; Fat: 13g; Sugar:0g; Sodium: 410mg; Fiber: 2.5g

Chocolate Chicken Mole

Serves: 6
Cook Time: 7 hours

Ingredients

- 2 pounds chicken pieces, skin and bones removed
- 2 tablespoons butter
- 1 onion, chopped
- 4 cloves of garlic, minced
- 7 tomatoes chopped
- 5 dried chili peppers, rehydrated then chopped
- ¼ cup organic and unsweetened almond butter
- ¼ cup unsweetened dark chocolate, shaved
- 1 teaspoon cumin powder
- ½ teaspoon cinnamon powder
- Salt and pepper to taste

Instructions

1. Place all ingredients in the CrockPot.
2. Close the lid and cook on high for 6 hours or on low for 7 hours.
3. Garnish with cilantro, avocado slices, lemon wedges, or sour cream.

Nutrition information: Calories per serving: 511; Carbohydrates: 5.2g; Protein: 46.8g; Fat: 30.9g; Sugar: 0g; Sodium: 1093mg; Fiber: 3.2g

Green Chili Chicken

Serves: 6
Cook Time: 8 hours

Ingredients

- 1 cup basil leaves
- ½ cup green chilies
- 2 tablespoon garlic salt
- 4 cloves of garlic
- 1 white onion, chopped
- 6 chicken thighs, bones and skin removed

Instructions

1. Place the basil, green chilies, garlic salt, garlic, and onion in a food processor. Pulse until smooth.
2. Place the chicken in the CrockPot and pour over the sauce.
3. Close the lid and cook on high for 6 hours or on low for 8 hours.

Nutrition information: Calories per serving: 436; Carbohydrates: 2.6g; Protein: 32.3g; Fat: 32.1g; Sugar: 0g; Sodium: 988mg; Fiber: 1.4g

CrockPot Salsa Chicken

Serves: 4
Cook Time: 7 hours

Ingredients

- 6 roma tomatoes, cut into quarters
- 1 jalapeno, seeded
- 1 yellow onion, quartered
- 3 cloves of garlic, peeled
- 1 cup cilantro leaves
- 1 teaspoon cumin
- 4 chicken breasts, skin and bones removed
- 2 tablespoons oil
- Salt and pepper to taste
- 2 tablespoon lime juice, freshly squeezed

Instructions

1. Place in a food processor tomatoes, jalapeno, onion, garlic, cilantro, and cumin. Pulse until smooth.
2. Place the chicken breasts in the CrockPot. Add in the oil and season with salt and pepper to taste.
3. Pour the homemade salsa and add in the lime juice.
4. Close the lid and cook on high for 5 hours or on low for 6 hours.

Nutrition information: Calories per serving: 598; Carbohydrates: 8.1g; Protein: g62.9; Fat: 34.2g; Sugar: 2.1g; Sodium: 1204mg; Fiber: 3.9g

CrockPot Tomato and Coconut Chicken

Serves: 6
Cook Time: 8 hours

Ingredients

- 2 pounds organic chicken thighs, bones and skin removed
- 1 onion, chopped
- 1 can full fat coconut milk, unsweetened
- 1 cup tomato, chopped and pureed
- 2 cloves of garlic, chopped
- 1 tablespoon red curry paste
- 2 ½ teaspoon yellow curry powder
- 1 teaspoon ginger, minced
- 1 teaspoon cumin
- ½ teaspoon garam masala
- ½ teaspoon cinnamon
- ¼ teaspoon cayenne pepper
- Salt and pepper to taste
- 1 bunch kale leaves, stems removed

Instructions

1. Place all ingredients except for the kale in the CrockPot.
2. Close the lid and cook on high for 5 hours or on low for 8 hours.
3. An hour before the cooking time ends, add in the kale leaves.
4. Continue cooking until the chicken is cooked through.

Nutrition information: Calories per serving: 462; Carbohydrates: 4.8g; Protein: 36.1g; Fat: 32.5g; Sugar: 0g; Sodium: 720mg; Fiber: 2.8g

Garlic Chipotle Lime Chicken

Serves: 6
Cook Time: 8 hours

Ingredients

- 1 ½ pounds chicken breasts, bones and skin removed
- ½ cup organic tomato sauce
- 2 tablespoons olive oil
- 2 cloves of garlic
- 2 tablespoons mild green chilies, chopped
- 1 tablespoon apple cider vinegar
- 3 tablespoons lime juice
- 1/3 cup fresh cilantro
- 1 ½ teaspoon chipotle pepper, chopped
- Salt and pepper to taste

Instructions

1. Place all ingredients in the CrockPot.
2. Close the lid and cook on high for 5 hours or on low for 8 hours.
3. Serve with lime wedges.

Nutrition information: Calories per serving:183; Carbohydrates: 2g; Protein: 22g; Fat: 9g; Sugar: 0g; Sodium: 527mg; Fiber: 1.2g

Mexican Chicken "Bake"

Serves: 6
Cook Time: 8 hours

Ingredients

- 6 roma tomatoes, cut into quarters
- 1 cup cilantro leaves
- 1 yellow onion, quartered
- 1 teaspoon cumin
- 1 jalapeno, seeded
- 3 cloves of garlic, peeled
- Salt and pepper to taste
- 2 pounds chicken breasts, bones and skin removed
- ½ cup queso quesadilla cheese, shredded
- 1-ounce black olives, pitted and sliced

Instructions

1. Place the tomatoes, cilantro, onion, cumin, jalapeno, and garlic in a food processor. Season with salt and pepper to taste. Pulse until smooth.
2. Place the chicken breasts in the CrockPot and pour over the salsa sauce.
3. Top with cheese and olives.
4. Close the lid and cook on high for 6 hours and on high for 8 hours.
5. Garnish with sour cream, avocado slices, or cilantro.

Nutrition information: Calories per serving: 203; Carbohydrates: 5g; Protein: 18g; Fat: 11g; Sugar: 0g; Sodium:637 mg; Fiber: 1g

Shredded Soy Lemon Chicken

Serves: 8
Cook Time: 8 hours

Ingredients

- 2 pounds chicken breasts, bones and skin removed
- 1 cup water
- ¼ cup lemon juice
- ½ cup soy sauce
- 4 cloves of garlic, minced
- 1 onion, chopped finely
- 2 tablespoons sesame oil
- Salt and pepper to taste

Instructions

1. Place all ingredients in the CrockPot.
2. Close the lid and cook on high for 6 hours or on low for 8 hours.
3. Once the chicken is very tender, shred the meat using two forks.
4. Serve with the sauce.

Nutrition information: Calories per serving: 283; Carbohydrates: 6.8g; Protein: 25.2g; Fat: 18.2g; Sugar: 1.2g; Sodium: 612mg; Fiber: 2.8g

CrockPot Rosemary Lemon Chicken

Serves: 6
Cook Time: 8 hours

Ingredients

- 1 tablespoon butter
- 4 pounds chicken breasts, bones and skin removed
- 3 onions, chopped
- 6 cloves of garlic, minced
- 3 sprigs of fresh rosemary
- ½ cup lemon juice, freshly squeezed
- ¾ cup homemade chicken broth
- 1 tablespoon lemon zest
- Salt and pepper to taste

Instructions

1. Place all ingredients in the CrockPot.
2. Close the lid and cook on high for 6 hours or on low for 8 hours.
3. Garnish with parsley.

Nutrition information: Calories per serving: 573; Carbohydrates: 4.8g; Protein: 64.3g; Fat: 30.1g; Sugar: 1.2g; Sodium: 837mg; Fiber: 2.7g

CrockPot Fajita Chicken

Serves: 8
Cook Time: 8 hours

Ingredients

- 2 ½ pounds chicken thighs and breasts, skin and bones removed
- 1 onion, sliced
- 4 cloves of garlic, minced
- 2 cups bell peppers, sliced
- 1 teaspoon ground coriander
- ½ teaspoon cumin
- ½ teaspoon chipotle pepper, chopped
- 1 cup roma tomatoes, diced
- Salt and pepper to taste

Instructions

1. Place all ingredients in the CrockPot.
2. Close the lid and cook on high for 6 hours or on low for 8 hours.
3. Shred the chicken meat using two forks.
4. Return to the CrockPot and cook on high for another 30 minutes.
5. Garnish with chopped cilantro.

Nutrition information: Calories per serving: 328; Carbohydrates: 3.3g; Protein: 39.5g; Fat: 17.7g; Sugar: 0g; Sodium: 697mg; Fiber: 1.7g

CrockPot Yellow Chicken Curry

Serves: 5
Cook Time: 8 hours

Ingredients

- 1 ½ pounds boneless chicken breasts, cut into chunks
- 6 cups vegetable broth (made from boiling onions, broccoli, bell pepper, and carrots in 7 cups water)
- 1 cup coconut milk, unsweetened
- 1 cup tomatoes, crushed
- 1 tablespoon cumin
- 2 teaspoons ground coriander
- 1 teaspoon turmeric powder
- 1 thumb-size ginger, sliced
- 4 cloves of garlic, minced
- 1 teaspoon cinnamon
- ½ teaspoon cayenne pepper
- Salt to taste

Instructions

1. Place all ingredients in the CrockPot.
2. Close the lid and cook on high for 6 hours or on low for 8 hours.

Nutrition information: Calories per serving: 291; Carbohydrates: 6.1g; Protein: 32.5g; Fat: 15.4g; Sugar: 0.3g; Sodium: 527mg; Fiber: 2.8g

Thai Clear Chicken Soup

Serves: 8
Cook Time: 8 hours

Ingredients

- 1 whole chicken, cut into pieces
- 1 stalk of lemon grass, cut into 5-inches in length
- 20 fresh basil leaves
- 5 slices of ginger
- Juice from 1 lime, freshly squeezed
- Salt and pepper to taste

Instructions

1. Place all ingredients in the CrockPot.
2. Close the lid and cook on high for 6 hours or on low for 8 hours.
3. Garnish with cilantro.

Nutrition information: Calories per serving: 236; Carbohydrates: 7.9g; Protein: 23.5g; Fat: 18.6g; Sugar: 0.8g; Sodium: 719mg; Fiber: 4.1g

Coconut Turmeric Chicken

Serves: 8
Cook Time: 8 hours

Ingredients

- 1 whole chicken, cut into pieces
- ½ cup coconut milk, unsweetened
- 2 inch-knob fresh turmeric, grated
- 2 inch-knob fresh ginger, grated
- 4 cloves of garlic, grated
- Salt and pepper to taste

Instructions

1. Place all ingredients in the CrockPot.
2. Close the lid and cook on high for 6 hours or on low for 8 hours.
3. Garnish with chopped scallions.

Nutrition information: Calories per serving: 270; Carbohydrates: 4.2g; Protein:24.5g; Fat: 18.9g; Sugar: 0g; Sodium: 883mg; Fiber: 1.6g

Turkey Soup with Rosemary and Kale

Serves: 6
Cook Time: 8 hours

Ingredients

- ½ onion, chopped
- 2 cloves of garlic, minced
- Salt and pepper to taste
- 1 tablespoon tallow or ghee
- 1-pound turkey meat, cut into bite-sized pieces
- 4 cups homemade chicken stock
- 2 sprigs rosemary, chopped
- 3 cups kale, chopped

Instructions

1. Place all ingredients except the kale in the CrockPot.
2. Close the lid and cook on high for 6 hours or on low for 8 hours.
3. An hour before the cooking time ends, add in the kale.
4. Close the lid and cook until the kale has wilted.

Nutrition information: Calories per serving: 867; Carbohydrates: 2.6g; Protein: 151.3g; Fat: 23.6g; Sugar: 0g; Sodium: 1373mg; Fiber: 1.4g

Chipotle Chicken Enchilada Stew

Serves: 5
Cook Time: 8 hours

Ingredients

- 1 ½ pounds chicken breasts, bones and skin removed
- 1 onion, chopped
- 1 green pepper, chopped
- 1 yellow pepper, chopped
- 3 jalapeno peppers, chopped
- 1 cup tomatoes, diced
- 2 cups homemade chicken stock
- 2 cups ground chicken
- 4 cloves of garlic, minced
- 1 tablespoon cumin
- 1 tablespoon chili powder
- 1 tablespoon chipotle pepper, chopped
- 1 teaspoon oregano
- Salt and pepper to taste

Instructions

1. Place all ingredients in the CrockPot.
2. Close the lid and cook on high for 6 hours or on low for 8 hours.
3. Serve with avocado slices and cilantro.

Nutrition information: Calories per serving: 708; Carbohydrates: 9.2g; Protein: 108.4g; Fat: 23.6g; Sugar: 0.8g; Sodium: 989mg; Fiber: 3.7g

Basic Shredded Chicken

Serves: 12
Cook Time: 8 hours

Ingredients

- 6 pounds chicken breasts, bones and skin removed
- 1 teaspoon salt
- ½ teaspoon black pepper
- 5 cups homemade chicken broth
- 4 tablespoons butter

Instructions

1. Place all ingredients in the CrockPot.
2. Close the lid and cook on high for 6 hours or on low for 8 hours.
3. Shred the chicken meat using two forks.
4. Return to the CrockPot and cook on high for another 30 minutes.

Nutrition information: Calories per serving: 421; Carbohydrates: 0.5g; Protein: 48.1g; Fat: 25.4g; Sugar: 0g; Sodium: 802mg; Fiber: 0.1g

Caribbean Pork Chop

Serves: 4
Preparation time: 3 minutes
Cooking time: 10 hours

Ingredients
- 1 tablespoon curry powder
- 1 teaspoon cumin
- Salt and pepper to taste
- 1-pound pork loin roast, bones removed
- ½ cup chicken broth

Instructions
1. Place all ingredients in the crockpot. Give a good stir.
2. Close the lid and cook on low for 8 to 10 hours or on high for 7 hours.

Nutrition information: Calories per serving: 471; Carbohydrates: 0.9g; Protein: 43.8g; Fat: 35g; Sugar: 0g; Sodium:528mg; Fiber: 0g

Crockpot Pork Roast

Serves: 4
Preparation time: 5 minutes
Cooking time: 12 hours

Ingredients
- 1-pound pork loin roast, bones removed
- 3 tablespoons olive oil
- 1 teaspoon thyme leaves
- 1 teaspoon marjoram leaves
- ½ tablespoon dry mustard

Instructions
1. Line the bottom of the crockpot with foil.
2. Combine all ingredients in a bowl. Massage the pork to coat all surface with the spices.
3. Place in the crockpot and cook on low for 12 hours or on high for 8 hours.

Nutrition information: Calories per serving: 414; Carbohydrates: 0.8g; Protein: 52.2; Fat: 37.1g; Sugar:0 g; Sodium: 724mg; Fiber: 0g

Pork Chops and Peppers

Serves: 4
Preparation time: 5 minutes
Cooking time: 10 hours

Ingredients
- 4 pork chops
- 1 onion, chopped
- 2 cups red and green bell peppers
- ½ cup chicken broth
- ½ teaspoon thyme leaves

Instructions
1. Place all ingredients in the crockpot.
2. Mix to combine all ingredients.
3. Close the lid and cook on low for 10 hours or on high for 7 hours.

Nutrition information: Calories per serving: 592; Carbohydrates: 0.5g; Protein: 47.1g; Fat: 39.2g; Sugar: 0g; Sodium:601 mg; Fiber:0 g

Italian Pork Chops

Serves: 6
Preparation time: 5 minutes
Cooking time: 10 hours

Ingredients
- 6 pork loin chops
- 1 onion, chopped
- 3 cloves of garlic, minced
- 3 cups sugar-free pasta sauce
- 1 cup mozzarella cheese

Instructions
1. Place pork loin, onion, and garlic in the crockpot.
2. Pour in the sugar-free pasta sauce.
3. Add the mozzarella cheese on top.
4. Close the lid and cook for low in 10 hours or on high for 7 hours.

Nutrition information: Calories per serving: 420; Carbohydrates: 6.2g; Protein: 38.1g; Fat: 29.4g; Sugar: 0.9g; Sodium: 672mg; Fiber: 3.4g

Easy Pork Chop Dinner

Serves: 4
Preparation time: 10 minutes
Cooking time: 10 hours

Ingredients

- 2 teaspoons olive oil
- 2 cloves of garlic, chopped
- 1 onion, chopped
- 4 pork cops
- 2 cups chicken broth

Instructions

1. In a skillet, heat the oil and sauté the garlic and onions until fragrant and lightly golden. Add in the pork chops and cook for 2 minutes for 2 minutes on each side.
2. Pour the chicken broth and scrape the bottom to remove the browning.
3. Transfer to the crockpot. Season with salt and pepper to taste.
4. Close the lid and cook on low for 10 hours or on high for 7 hours.

Nutrition information: Calories per serving: 481; Carbohydrates: 2.5g; Protein: 38.1g; Fat: 30.5g; Sugar: 0.3g; Sodium: 735mg; Fiber: 1.2g

Cheesy Pork Casserole

Serves: 4
Preparation time: 5 minutes
Cooking time: 10 hours

Ingredients

- 4 pork chops, bones removed and sliced
- 1 cauliflower head, cut into florets
- 1 cup chicken broth
- 1 teaspoon rosemary
- 2 cups cheddar cheese

Instructions

1. Arrange the pork chop slices in the crockpot,
2. Add in the cauliflower florets.
3. Pour the chicken broth and rosemary. Season with salt and pepper to taste.
4. Pour cheddar cheese on top.
5. Close the lid and cook on low for 10 hours.

Nutrition information: Calories per serving: 417; Carbohydrates: 7g; Protein: 32.1g; Fat: 26.2g; Sugar: 0; Sodium: 846mg; Fiber: 5.3g

One Pot Pork Chops

Serves: 6
Preparation time: 3 minutes
Cooking time: 10 hours

Ingredients
- 6 pork chops
- 2 cups broccoli florets
- ½ cup green and red bell peppers
- 1 onion, sliced
- Salt and pepper to taste

Instructions
1. Place all ingredients in the crockpot.
2. Give a stir to mix everything.
3. Close the lid and cook on low for 10 hours or on high for 8 hours.

Nutrition information: Calories per serving: 496; Carbohydrates: 6g; Protein: 37.1g; Fat: 23.7g; Sugar: 0.8g; Sodium: 563mg; Fiber: 4.3g

Easy Crockpot Pulled Pork

Serves: 4
Preparation time: 3 minutes
Cooking time: 12 hours

Ingredients
- 4 pork shoulder, trimmed from excess fat
- 1 small onion, sliced
- Salt and pepper to taste
- 1 cup water
- 1 teaspoon rosemary

Instructions
1. Place all ingredients in the crockpot.
2. Cook on low for 12 hours or on high for 8 hours.
3. Once cooked, use forks to shred the meat.

Nutrition information: Calories per serving: 533; Carbohydrates: 2g; Protein: 47.2g; Fat: 32.3g; Sugar: 0g; Sodium: 629mg; Fiber: 1.4g

Jalapeno Basil Pork Chops

Serves: 4
Preparation time: 3 minutes
Cooking time: 12 hours

Ingredients
- ½ cup jalapeno peppers, chopped
- 4 pork loin, chopped
- ½ cup dry white wine
- ¼ cup fresh basil
- Salt and pepper to taste

Instructions
1. Place all ingredients in the crockpot.
2. Give a good stir to combine all ingredients.
3. Cook on low for 12 hours or on high for 8 hours.

Nutrition information: Calories per serving: 472; Carbohydrates: 6.1g; Protein: 38.2g; Fat:29.1 g; Sugar: 0.6g; Sodium: 723mg; Fiber: 4.3g

Bacon-Wrapped Pork Tenderloin

Serves: 4
Preparation time: 5 minutes
Cooking time: 10 hours

Ingredients
- 1-pound pork tenderloin
- Salt and pepper to taste
- 1 teaspoon rosemary leaves
- 3 bacon slices, cut in half lengthwise
- 2 tablespoons butter, melted

Instructions
1. Season the pork tenderloin with salt and pepper to taste.
2. Sprinkle with rosemary and massage the pork.
3. Arrange bacon slices all over the pork.
4. Brush melted butter all over.
5. Place in the crockpot and cook on low for 10 hours or on high for 8 hours.

Nutrition information: Calories per serving: 401; Carbohydrates: 1g; Protein: 38.5g; Fat: 34.1g; Sugar: 0g; Sodium: 623mg; Fiber: 0.7g

Crockpot Pork Adobo

Serves: 2
Preparation time: 3 minutes
Cooking time: 12 hours

Ingredients
- ¼ cup Soy Sauce
- 4 tablespoons apple cider vinegar
- 1-pound pork loin, chopped
- 1 bay leaf
- 1 teaspoon whole peppercorns

Instructions
1. Place all ingredients in the crockpot.
2. Give a good stir to combine all ingredients.
3. Cook on low for 12 hours or on high for 8 hours.

Nutrition information: Calories per serving: 328; Carbohydrates: 3.21g; Protein: 53.84g; Fat: 9.38g; Sugar: 0.29g; Sodium: 1261mg; Fiber: 0.7g

Dijon Basil Pork Loin

Serves: 4
Preparation time: 7 minutes
Cooking time: 10 hours

Ingredients
- 1 pork loin roast, trimmed from excess fat
- 2 tablespoons Dijon mustard
- 1 teaspoon marjoram
- Salt and pepper to taste
- ¼ cup basil, chopped

Instructions
1. Rub the pork loin roast with mustard, marjoram, salt and pepper.
2. Use your hands to massage the pork.
3. Place in the crockpot and sprinkle with chopped basil.
4. Close the lid and cook on low for 10 hours or on high for 8 hours.

Nutrition information: Calories per serving: 449; Carbohydrates: 3g; Protein: 38.2g; Fat:33.1g; Sugar:0 g; Sodium: 764mg; Fiber: 1.3g

Bacon Swiss Pork Chops

Serves: 8
Preparation time: 10 minutes
Cooking time: 10 hours

Ingredients
- 8 pork chops, bone in
- 2 tablespoons olive oil
- 1 cup Swiss cheese, shredded
- 4 cloves of garlic
- 12 bacon strips, cut in half

Instructions
1. Season the pork chops with salt and pepper to taste
2. In a skillet, heat the olive oil over medium flame and sauté the garlic until fragrant and slightly golden.
3. Transfer to the crockpot.
4. Wrap the bacon strips around the pork chops.
5. Place in the crockpot and sprinkle with shredded Swiss cheese.
6. Close the lid and cook on low for 10 hours or on high for 8 hours.

Nutrition information: Calories per serving: 519; Carbohydrates: 0.5g; Protein: 42.3g; Fat: 40.2g; Sugar: 0g; Sodium: 732mg; Fiber: 0g

Mole Pork Chops

Serves: 3
Preparation time: 3 minutes
Cooking time: 10 hours

Ingredients
- 1 tablespoon butter, melted
- 3 pork chops, bone in
- 2 teaspoons paprika
- ½ teaspoon cocoa powder, unsweetened
- Salt and pepper to taste

Instructions
1. Place the butter into the crockpot.
2. Season the pork chops with paprika, cocoa powder, salt and pepper.
3. Arrange in the crockpot.
4. Close the lid and cook on low for 10 hours or on high for 8 hours.
5. Halfway through the cooking time, be sure to flip the pork chops.

Nutrition information: Calories per serving: 579; Carbohydrates: 1.2g; Protein: 41.7g; Fat: 34.7g; Sugar: 0g; Sodium: 753mg; Fiber: 0g

Simple Pork Chop Casserole

Serves: 4
Preparation time: 3 minutes
Cooking time: 10 hours

Ingredients
- 4 pork chops, bones removed and cut into bite-sized pieces
- 3 tablespoons minced onion
- ½ cup water
- Salt and pepper to taste
- 1 cup heavy cream

Instructions
1. Place the pork chop slices, onions, and water in the crockpot.
2. Season with salt and pepper to taste.
3. Close the lid and cook on low for 10 hours or on high for 8 hours.
4. Halfway through the cooking time, pour in the heavy cream.

Nutrition information: Calories per serving: 515; Carbohydrates: 2.5g; Protein: 39.2g; Fat: 34.3g; Sugar: 0g; Sodium: 613mg; Fiber:0.9 g

Crockpot Pulled Pork

Serves: 4
Preparation time: 3 minutes
Cooking time: 12 hours

Ingredients
- 2 onions, cut into slices
- 1-pound pork shoulder roast, bones removed
- 2 tablespoons garlic powder
- Salt and pepper to taste
- 2 cups chicken broth

Instructions
1. Place all ingredients in the crockpot.
2. Close the lid and cook on low for 12 hours or on high for 10 hours.
3. Once cooked, take the meat out from the crockpot and shred using two forks.
4. Place the shredded meat back into the crockpot and allow to simmer for another two hours or until the meat is soaked in its juices.

Nutrition information: Calories per serving:492; Carbohydrates: 1g; Protein: 36.1g; Fat: 29.5g; Sugar:0 g; Sodium:524 mg; Fiber: 0.7g

Chinese Pork Ribs

Serves: 6
Preparation time: 3 minutes
Cooking time: 12 hours

Ingredients
- ¼ cup soy sauce
- 2 cloves of garlic
- 2 tablespoons Chinese five-spice powder
- 4 pounds pork ribs, bone in
- 3 tablespoons sugar-free ketchup

Instructions
1. Combine everything in the crockpot.
2. Close the lid and cook on low for 12 hours or on high for 8 hours.

Nutrition information: Calories per serving: 373; Carbohydrates: 4g; Protein:27 g; Fat:14g; Sugar: 2.1g; Sodium: 562mg; Fiber: 0g

Pork Roast in Crockpot

Serves: 8
Preparation time: 3 minutes
Cooking time: 12 hours

Ingredients
- 3 pounds pork shoulder roast
- 2 tablespoons herb mix of your choice
- 1 cup onion, chopped
- Salt and pepper to taste
- 2 cups chicken broth

Instructions
1. Combine everything in the crockpot.
2. Close the lid and cook on low for 12 hours or on high for 8 hours.

Nutrition information: Calories per serving: 408; Carbohydrates: 2.73g; Protein: 41.92g; Fat: 24.53g; Sugar: 0.89g; Sodium: 382mg; Fiber: 0.7g

Ginger and Rosemary Pork Ribs

Serves: 4
Preparation time: 3 minutes
Cooking time: 12 hours

Ingredients
- 1/3 cup chicken broth
- 4 racks pork spare ribs
- 3 tablespoons ginger paste or powder
- 1 teaspoon rosemary, dried
- Salt and pepper to taste

Instructions
1. Pour the broth into the crockpot.
2. Season the spare ribs with ginger paste, rosemary, salt and pepper.
3. Place in the crockpot.
4. Close the lid and cook on low for 12 hours or on high for 8 hours.

Nutrition information: Calories per serving: 396; Carbohydrates: 03g; Protein: 27.1g; Fat: 21g; Sugar: 0g; Sodium: 582mg; Fiber: 0g

Baked Pork Chops

Serves: 4
Preparation time: 5 minutes
Cooking time: 12 hours

Ingredients
- 4 pork chops, bone in
- 2 teaspoons olive oil
- 1 ½ tablespoons herbes de Provence
- Salt and pepper to taste
- 2 tablespoons parsley, chopped

Instructions
1. Season the pork chops with herbs, salt and pepper.
2. Brush the pork chops with oil.
3. Place in the crockpot that has been lined with foil.
4. Sprinkle with parsley.
5. Close the lid and cook on high for 8 hours or on low for 12 hours.

Nutrition information: Calories per serving: 481; Carbohydrates:0.4 g; Protein: 37.2g; Fat: 25.8g; Sugar: 0g; Sodium: 471mg; Fiber:0 g

Pork Stew with Oyster Mushrooms

Serves: 8
Cook Time:

Ingredients

- 2 tablespoons coconut oil
- 1 onion, chopped
- 1 clove of garlic, minced
- 2 pounds pork loin cut into cubes
- 3 tablespoons dried oregano
- 2 tablespoons dried mustard
- 1 ½ cups bone broth
- 2 pounds oyster mushrooms, minced
- ¼ cup coconut milk
- 3 tablespoons capers
- Salt and pepper to taste

Instructions

1. Place all ingredients in the CrockPot.
2. Give a good stir.
3. Close the lid and cook on high for 8 hours or on low for 10 hours.

Nutrition information: Calories per serving: 734; Carbohydrates:4.2 g; Protein: 50.4g; Fat: 48.9g; Sugar: 0g; Sodium: 1118mg; Fiber: 2.6g

CrockPot Pork Shanks

Serves: 10
Cook Time: 10 hours

Ingredients

- 1 ½ tablespoons avocado oil
- 3 pounds pork shanks, bone-in
- 3 cups onion, chopped
- 4 cloves of garlic, minced
- 3 cups mushrooms, chopped
- 1 tablespoon oregano leaves, minced
- 2 teaspoons thyme leaves
- 2 tablespoons basil leaves, finely
- ¾ cup chicken broth
- Salt and pepper to taste

Instructions

1. Place all ingredients in the CrockPot.
2. Give a good stir.
3. Close the lid and cook on high for 8 hours or on low for 10 hours.

Nutrition information: Calories per serving: 233; Carbohydrates: 5.2g; Protein: 34.8g; Fat: 7.5g; Sugar: 0g; Sodium: 811mg; Fiber: 2.5g

CrockPot Pork Chili Verde

Serves: 9
Cook Time: 10 hours

Ingredients

- 1 cup tomatoes, chopped
- 1 cup onions, quartered
- 4 cloves of garlic, chopped
- 2 green chili peppers
- ½ teaspoon oregano
- ½ teaspoon cumin
- 2 pounds pork stew meat, bones removed
- 3 tablespoons butter, melted
- 3 tablespoons cilantro, chopped

Instructions

1. In a blender, place the tomatoes, onions, garlic, chili peppers, oregano, and cumin. Blend until smooth.
2. Pour into the CrockPot and add the meat and butter.
3. Close the lid and cook on high for 8 hours or on low for 10 hours.
4. Garnish with cilantro once cooked.

Nutrition information: Calories per serving: 307; Carbohydrates: 4.6g; Protein: 29g; Fat: 16g; Sugar: 0g; Sodium: 529mg; Fiber: 4g

Pork Loin Roast in CrockPot

Serves: 8
Cook Time: 12 hours

Ingredients

- 2 pounds pork loin
- 2 onions, chopped
- 3 cups homemade beef stock
- Salt and pepper to taste

Instructions

1. Place all ingredients in the CrockPot.
2. Give a good stir.
3. Close the lid and cook on high for 10 hours or on low for 12 hours.

Nutrition information: Calories per serving: 282; Carbohydrates: 4.7g; Protein: 30.6g; Fat: 15.9g; Sugar: 0g; Sodium: 635mg; Fiber: 2.8g

Italian Pork Roast

Serves: 10
Cook Time: 12 hours

Ingredients

- 5 pounds pork shoulder, bone in
- 7 cloves of garlic, slivered
- 1 tablespoon salt
- 1 teaspoon dried oregano
- 1 teaspoon dried basil
- 1 teaspoon dried rosemary
- ½ teaspoon black pepper

Instructions

1. Place all ingredients in the CrockPot.
2. Give a good stir.
3. Close the lid and cook on high for 10 hours or on low for 12 hours.

Nutrition information: Calories per serving: 610; Carbohydrates: 0.9g; Protein: 57.1g; Fat: 40.8g; Sugar: 0g; Sodium: 1240mg; Fiber: 0.2g

Mexican Carne Adovada

Serves: 9
Cook Time: 12 hours

Ingredients

- 3 pounds pork Boston butt
- 2 dried chili peppers, chopped
- 2 ancho peppers, chopped
- 2 guajillo peppers, chopped
- 2 cups homemade beef stock
- 1 onion, chopped
- 6 cloves of garlic, minced
- 1 teaspoon cumin
- 1 teaspoon coriander
- 2 teaspoons apple cider vinegar
- Salt and pepper to taste

Instructions

1. Place all ingredients in the CrockPot.
2. Give a good stir.
3. Close the lid and cook on high for 10 hours or on low for 12 hours.

Nutrition information: Calories per serving: 453; Carbohydrates: 4.8; Protein: 39.9g; Fat: 28.1g; Sugar: 0.3g; Sodium: 991mg; Fiber: 2.4g

5-Spice CrockPot Pork Ribs

Serves: 8
Cook Time: 12 hours

Ingredients

- 4 pounds baby back ribs
- 2 teaspoons Chinese five-spice powder
- ¾ teaspoon garlic powder
- 1 jalapeno pepper, cut into rings
- 2 tablespoons rice vinegar
- 2 tablespoons coconut aminos
- 1 tablespoon organic tomato paste
- Salt and pepper to taste

Instructions

1. Place all ingredients in the CrockPot.
2. Give a good stir.
3. Close the lid and cook on high for 10 hours or on low for 12 hours.

Nutrition information: Calories per serving: 508; Carbohydrates:1.8 g; Protein: 45g; Fat: 35.7g; Sugar: 0g; Sodium: 840mg; Fiber: 0.7g

CrockPot Scotch Eggs

Serves: 8
Cook Time: 12 hours

Ingredients

- 2 tablespoons olive oil
- 2 pounds ground pork
- 2 teaspoons salt
- 1 teaspoon ground black pepper
- ½ teaspoon nutmeg
- 1 teaspoon cloves
- ¼ cup parsley leaves, minced
- 2 cloves of garlic, minced
- 2 large eggs, raw
- 8 large eggs, boiled and peeled

Instructions

1. Line the CrockPot with aluminum foil. Grease with olive oil.
2. In a mixing bowl, mix all ingredients except for the boiled eggs.
3. Form balls with the meat mixture and flatten using the palm of your palms. Add the boiled eggs in the center and fold the meat over the eggs to form one large meatball.
4. Place the scotch eggs in the CrockPot.
5. Close the lid and cook on high for 8 hours or on high for 12 hours.

Nutrition information: Calories per serving:463; Carbohydrates: 1.7g; Protein:36.3 g; Fat: 33.4g; Sugar: 0g; Sodium: 926mg; Fiber: 0.8g

CrockPot Polish Hunter's Stew

Serves: 8
Cook Time: 12 hours

Ingredients

- ½ ounce porcini mushrooms, sliced
- 2 pounds pork stew meat, bones removed
- ½ pound smoked nitrate-free sausages, chopped
- 2 onions, diced
- 1 teaspoon caraway seeds
- 2 bay leaves
- 1 cup tomatoes, chopped
- 6 cups beef stock
- Salt and pepper to taste

Instructions

1. Place all ingredients in the CrockPot.
2. Give a good stir.
3. Close the lid and cook on high for 10 hours or on low for 12 hours.

Nutrition information: Calories per serving: 312; Carbohydrates: 5.4g; Protein: 42.8g; Fat: 15.5g; Sugar: 0g; Sodium: 711mg; Fiber: 3.2g

Garlic Pork Stew

Serves: 4
Cook Time: 10 hours

Ingredients

- 1 tablespoon coconut oil
- 1-pound pork shoulder, cut into cubes
- 1 onion, diced
- 8 cloves of garlic, minced
- 2 cups homemade chicken broth
- 2 tablespoons mustard
- Salt and pepper to taste

Instructions

1. Place all ingredients in the CrockPot.
2. Give a good stir.
3. Close the lid and cook on high for 8 hours or on low for 10 hours.

Nutrition information: Calories per serving: 369; Carbohydrates: 4.6g; Protein: 30.4g; Fat: 24.9g; Sugar: 0g; Sodium: 731mg; Fiber: 2.1g

CrockPot Pork Carnitas

Serves: 12
Cook Time: 12 hours

Ingredients

- 4 pounds pork shoulder
- ½ cup lime juice, freshly squeezed
- ½ cup lemon juice, freshly squeezed
- 1 tablespoon ground cumin
- 1 tablespoon garlic powder
- ½ tablespoon salt
- 1 teaspoon ground coriander
- 1 teaspoon black pepper
- 1 teaspoon cayenne pepper

Instructions

1. Place all ingredients in the CrockPot.
2. Give a good stir.
3. Close the lid and cook on high for 10 hours or on low for 12 hours.
4. Once cooked, shred the meat using two forks.

Nutrition information: Calories per serving:414; Carbohydrates: 2.8g; Protein:38.3 g; Fat: 29.6g; Sugar: 0g; Sodium: 815mg; Fiber: 1.6g

Spiced Pork Belly

Serves: 8
Cook Time: 12 hours

Ingredients

- 1 tablespoon olive oil
- 2-pound pork belly
- 3 cloves of garlic, crushed
- ½ teaspoon ground black pepper
- ½ teaspoon turmeric
- ½ teaspoon ground cumin
- ½ tablespoon lemon juice
- ½ tablespoon salt

Instructions

1. Line the bottom of the CrockPot with aluminum foil. Grease the foil with olive oil.
2. Place all ingredients in a mixing bowl. Massage and allow to marinate in the fridge for 2 hours.
3. Place inside the CrockPot.
4. Close the lid and cook on high for 10 hours or on low for 12 hours.

Nutrition information: Calories per serving: 606; Carbohydrates: 0.9g; Protein: 30.8g; Fat: 29.3g; Sugar: 0g; Sodium: 1007mg; Fiber: 0.4g

Simple CrockPot Meatballs

Serves: 4
Cook Time: 10 hours

Ingredients

- 2 tablespoons olive oil
- 2 tablespoons almonds, slivered
- 1-pound ground pork
- 1 tablespoon organic tomato paste
- 2 cloves of garlic, minced
- 1 teaspoon salt
- 1 teaspoon ground cinnamon
- ½ teaspoon dried oregano leaves
- ¼ teaspoon ground black pepper
- 2 tablespoons warm water
- ¼ teaspoon baking soda

Instructions

1. Line the bottom of the CrockPot with aluminum foil. Grease the foil with olive oil.
2. Place all ingredients in a mixing bowl. Form small meatballs using your hands.
3. Place in the CrockPot.
4. Close the lid and cook on high for 8 hours or on low for 10 hours.
5. Halfway through the cooking time, flip the meatballs to brown the other side.
6. Close the lid and continue cooking until the meat is cooked through.

Nutrition information: Calories per serving:407; Carbohydrates: 1.9g; Protein: 29.6g; Fat: 30.7g; Sugar: 0g; Sodium: 825mg; Fiber:0.6g

Fiesta Pork Chops

Serves: 4
Cook Time: 12 hours

Ingredients

- 4 large pork chops, bone in
- Salt and pepper to taste
- ½ tablespoons ghee
- ½ onion, diced
- 2 cloves of garlic, minced
- 1 teaspoon chili powder
- ¼ teaspoon oregano leaves
- 2/3 cup homemade chicken broth
- 1 tablespoon lime juice
- 1/8 cup mild green chilies, diced
- Salt and pepper to taste
- ¼ cup fresh cilantro, chopped

Instructions

1. Place all ingredients except the cilantro in the CrockPot.
2. Give a good stir.
3. Close the lid and cook on high for 10 hours or on low for 12 hours.
4. Garnish with cilantro once cooked.

Nutrition information: Calories per serving: 365; Carbohydrates: 5.1g; Protein: 41.3g; Fat: 19.1g; Sugar: 0g; Sodium: 720mg; Fiber:3.5g

CrockPot Gingered Pork Stew

Serves: 9
Cook Time: 12 hours

Ingredients

- 2 tablespoons ground cinnamon
- 2 tablespoons ground ginger
- 1 tablespoon ground allspice
- 1 tablespoon ground nutmeg
- 1 ½ teaspoons ground cloves
- 1 tablespoon paprika
- 3 pounds pork shoulder, cut into cubes
- 2 cups homemade chicken broth
- Salt and pepper to taste

Instructions

1. Place all ingredients in the CrockPot.
2. Give a good stir.
3. Close the lid and cook on high for 10 hours or on low for 12 hours.

Nutrition information: Calories per serving: 425; Carbohydrates: 4.2g; Protein: 38.7g; Fat: 27.4g; Sugar: 0g; Sodium: 803mg; Fiber: 2.8g

Classic Pork Adobo

Serves: 6
Cook Time: 12 hours

Ingredients

- 2 pounds pork chops, sliced
- 4 cloves of garlic, minced
- 1 onion, chopped
- 2 bay leaves
- ¼ cup soy sauce
- ½ cup lemon juice, freshly squeezed
- 4 quail eggs, boiled and peeled

Instructions

1. Place all ingredients except the quail eggs in the CrockPot.
2. Give a good stir.
3. Close the lid and cook on high for 10 hours or on low for 12 hours.
4. Add in quail eggs an hour before the cooking time ends.

Nutrition information: Calories per serving: 371; Carbohydrates: 6.4g; Protein: 40.7g; Fat: 24.1g; Sugar: 0g; Sodium: 720mg; Fiber: 3.9g

Herb-Crusted Pork Chops

Serves: 4
Cook Time: 12 hours

Ingredients

- 1 teaspoon parsley flakes
- 1 teaspoon dried marjoram
- ½ teaspoon ground thyme
- 1/8 teaspoon salt
- 1/8 teaspoon black pepper
- 2 tablespoons olive oil
- 4 pork chops
- ½ cup chicken broth

Instructions

1. Place all ingredients in the CrockPot.
2. Give a good stir.
3. Close the lid and cook on high for 10 hours or on low for 12 hours.

Nutrition information: Calories per serving: 436; Carbohydrates: 0.4g; Protein: 46.7g; Fat: 26.2g; Sugar: 0g; Sodium: 591mg; Fiber: 0.1g

Spicy Pork with Mapo Tofu

Serves: 2
Cook Time: 8 hours

Ingredients

- 2 tablespoons vegetable oil
- 8 ounces ground pork
- 1 jalapeno, sliced
- 4 garlic cloves, sliced
- 1 ½-inch ginger, grated
- 1 tablespoon tomato paste
- 1 teaspoon Sichuan peppercorns
- 2 cups chicken broth
- 1-pound silken tofu, drained and cubed

Instructions

1. Heat the oil in skillet over medium flame and render the ground pork for 3 minutes while stirring constantly.
2. Transfer the meat into the CrockPot then place all ingredients except for the silken tofu.
3. Give a good stir.
4. Close the lid and cook on high for 6 hours or on low for 8 hours.
5. An hour before the cooking time ends, add in the tofu cubes.

Nutrition information: Calories per serving:372; Carbohydrates: 5.3g; Protein:30.3 g; Fat: 25.8g; Sugar: 0.2g; Sodium: 756mg; Fiber: 2.4g

Herbed Pork Tenderloin

Serves: 6
Cook Time: 12 hours

Ingredients

- 2 pork tenderloins, skin removed
- ½ cup extra virgin olive oil
- ½ cup apple cider vinegar
- ½ cup cilantro, chopped
- 3 green onions, chopped
- 2 jalapeno peppers, chopped
- 2 tablespoons ginger, grated
- 1 teaspoon salt
- ½ teaspoon ground black pepper
- ½ teaspoon all spice
- 1/8 teaspoon ground cloves

Instructions

1. Mix all ingredients in a bowl and allow meat to marinate in the fridge for at least 2 hours.
2. Line aluminum foil at the base of the CrockPot.
3. Place the meat.
4. Close the lid and cook on high for 10 hours or on low for 12 hours.

Nutrition information: Calories per serving: 253; Carbohydrates: 5.5g; Protein: 29.8g; Fat: 13.6g; Sugar: 0.3g; Sodium: 739mg; Fiber:2.8 g

CrockPot Creamy Pork Chops

Serves: 9
Cook Time: 12 hours

Ingredients

- 3 tablespoons olive oil
- 9 boneless pork chops
- 1 tablespoon salt
- 1 teaspoon garlic powder
- 1 ½ teaspoons ground mustard
- 2 cups full-fat milk, unsweetened

Instructions

1. Place all ingredients in the CrockPot.
2. Give a good stir.
3. Close the lid and cook on high for 10 hours or on low for 12 hours.

Nutrition information: Calories per serving: 511; Carbohydrates: 2g; Protein: 25g; Fat: 43g; Sugar: 0g; Sodium: 617mg; Fiber: 0g

Chapter 6: Beef and Lamb Recipes

Skirt Steak with Red Pepper Sauce

Serves: 4
Preparation time: 12 minutes
Cooking time: 12 hours

Ingredients
- 2 red bell peppers, chopped
- 2 tablespoons olive oil
- 1 teaspoon thyme leaves
- 1-pound skirt steak, sliced into 1 inch thick
- Salt and pepper to taste

Instructions
1. In a food processor, mix together the red bell peppers, olive oil, and thyme leaves. Blend until smooth. Add water to make the mixture slightly runny. Set aside.
2. Season the skirt steak with salt and pepper.
3. Place in the crockpot and pour over the pepper sauce.
4. Add more salt and pepper if desired.
5. Close the lid and cook on low for 12 hours or on high for 10 hours.

Nutrition information: Calories per serving: 396; Carbohydrates:4 g; Protein: 32.5g; Fat: 21g; Sugar: 0g; Sodium: 428mg; Fiber: 2.8g

Beef Pot Roast

Serves: 6
Preparation time: 3 minutes
Cooking time: 12 hours

Ingredients
- 2 pounds shoulder pot roast, bones removed
- Salt and pepper to taste
- ¼ cup water
- 1 package mushrooms, sliced
- 1 tablespoon Worcestershire sauce

Instructions
1. Place all ingredients in the crockpot.
2. Give a good stir.
3. Close the lid and cook on low for 12 hours or on high for 10 hours.

Nutrition information: Calories per serving: 419; Carbohydrates:3 g; Protein: 32.6g; Fat: 29.6g; Sugar: 0.7g; Sodium: 513mg; Fiber: 1.4g

Smothered Pepper Steak

Serves: 4
Preparation time: 5 minutes
Cooking time: 10 hours

Ingredients
- 1 can diced tomatoes
- 1 package bell peppers
- Salt and pepper to taste
- 1 tablespoon soy sauce
- 4 sirloin patties

Instructions
1. Place the diced tomatoes (juices and all) in the crockpot.
2. Add the bell peppers. Season with salt, pepper, and soy sauce.
3. Arrange the sirloin patties on top.
4. Close the lid and cook on low for 10 hours or on high for 7 hours.

Nutrition information: Calories per serving: 387; Carbohydrates: 5g; Protein: 24.1g; Fat: 18.5g; Sugar: 0.8g; Sodium: 462mg; Fiber: 2.7g

Tenderloin Steaks with Red Wine and Mushrooms

Serves: 4
Preparation time: 3 minutes
Cooking time: 12 hours

Ingredients
- 4 pounds beef tenderloin steaks
- Salt and pepper to taste
- 1 package Portobello mushrooms, sliced
- 1 cup dry red wine
- 2 tablespoons butter

Instructions
1. Place all ingredients in the crockpot.
2. Give a good stir.
3. Close the lid and cook on low for 12 hours or on high for 10 hours.

Nutrition information: Calories per serving: 415; Carbohydrates:7.2 g; Protein:30.3 g; Fat: 27.4g; Sugar: 0g; Sodium: 426mg; Fiber:3.8 g

Naked Beef Enchilada in A Crockpot

Serves: 4
Preparation time: 8 minutes
Cooking time: 6 hours

Ingredients
- 1-pound ground beef
- 2 tablespoons enchilada spice mix
- 1 cup cauliflower florets
- 2 cups Mexican cheese blend, grated
- ¼ cup cilantro, chopped

Instructions
1. In a skillet, sauté the ground beef over medium flame for 3 minutes.
2. Transfer to the crockpot and add the enchilada spice mix and cauliflower.
3. Stir to combine.
4. Add the Mexican cheese blend on top.
5. Cook on low for 6 hours or on high for 4 hours.
6. Sprinkle with cilantro on top.

Nutrition information: Calories per serving: 481; Carbohydrates: 1g; Protein: 35.1g; Fat: 29.4g; Sugar: 0g; Sodium: 536mg; Fiber:0 g

Crockpot Cheeseburgers Casserole

Serves: 4
Preparation time: 10 minutes
Cooking time: 8 hours

Ingredients
- 1 white onion, chopped
- 1 ½ pounds lean ground beef
- 2 tablespoons mustard
- 1 teaspoon dried basil leaves
- 2 cups cheddar cheese

Instructions
1. Heat skillet over medium flame and sauté both white onions and ground beef for 3 minutes. Continue stirring until lightly brown.
2. Transfer to the crockpot and stir in mustard and basil leaves. Season with salt and pepper.
3. Add cheese on top.
4. Close the lid and cook on low for 8 hours and on high for 6 hours.

Nutrition information: Calories per serving: 472; Carbohydrates: 3g; Protein: 32.7g; Fat: 26.2g; Sugar: 0g; Sodium: 429mg; Fiber: 2.4g

Chili Crockpot Brisket

Serves: 4
Preparation time: 3 minutes
Cooking time: 12 hours

Ingredients
- 4 pounds beef brisket
- 1 bottle chili sauce
- Salt and pepper to taste
- 1 cup onion, chopped
- 1/8 cup water

Instructions
1. Place all ingredients in the crockpot.
2. Give a good stir.
3. Close the lid and cook on low for 12 hours or on high for 10 hours.

Nutrition information: Calories per serving: 634; Carbohydrates: 2.1g; Protein: 30.2g; Fat: 45.4g; Sugar:0 g; Sodium: 835mg; Fiber: 1.4g

Simple Roast Beef

Serves: 4
Preparation time: 3 minutes
Cooking time: 12 hours

Ingredients
- 2 pounds rump roast
- 1 cup onion, chopped
- 3 tablespoons butter
- Salt and pepper to taste
- ¼ cup water

Instructions
1. Place all ingredients in the crockpot.
2. Give a good stir.
3. Close the lid and cook on low for 12 hours or on high for 10 hours.
4. Once cooked, shred the pot roast using two forks.
5. Return to the crockpot and continue cooking on high for 1 hour.

Nutrition information: Calories per serving: 523; Carbohydrates:1.8g; Protein: 43.6g; Fat: 32.6g; Sugar: 0g; Sodium: 734mg; Fiber:1.2 g

Crockpot Beef and Broccoli

Serves: 2
Preparation time: 10 minutes
Cooking time: 12 hours

Ingredients

- ½ stick butter
- 2 tablespoons garlic, minced
- 2 cups stir fry beef
- 1 broccoli head, cut into florets
- ½ cup parmesan cheese, grated

Instructions

1. Heat oil in a skillet over medium flame and sauté the garlic until fragrant and lightly brown.
2. Add the beef and stir fry for 3 minutes. Stir constantly.
3. Transfer to the crockpot and add the broccoli florets. Season with salt and pepper to taste.
4. Add a few tablespoons of water.
5. Pour the parmesan cheese on top.
6. Close the lid and cook on low for 12 hours or on high for 9 hours.

Nutrition information: Calories per serving: 427; Carbohydrates: 0.9g; Protein: 34.2g; Fat: 32.7g; Sugar: 0g; Sodium:617 mg; Fiber: 0g

Roasted Beef Tenderloin

Serves: 5
Preparation time: 10 minutes
Cooking time: 12 hours

Ingredients

- 3 ½ pounds beef tenderloin
- Salt and pepper to taste
- 1 teaspoon dry mustard
- 3 tablespoons unsalted butter
- 2 cloves of garlic, minced

Instructions

1. Line the bottom of the crockpot with foil.
2. Season the beef tenderloin with salt and pepper. Rub the dry mustard.
3. In a skillet, heat the butter over medium flame. Sauté the garlic until lightly brown and fragrant.
4. Sear the beef tenderloin in the skillet for 2 minutes on each side.
5. Place in the crockpot.
6. Close the lid and cook on low for 12 hours or on high for 9 hours.

Nutrition information: Calories per serving: 473; Carbohydrates: 0.7g; Protein: 32.5g; Fat: 24.1g; Sugar: 0g; Sodium: 527mg; Fiber: 0g

Soy Beef Steak

Serves: 4
Preparation time: 3 minutes
Cooking time: 12 hours

Ingredients
- 2 pounds beef tenderloin, sliced thinly
- ¼ cup soy sauce
- ¼ cup lemon juice
- 1 bay leaf
- 1 large red onion, sliced into rings

Instructions
1. Place all ingredients in the crockpot.
2. Give a good stir.
3. Close the lid and cook on low for 12 hours or on high for 10 hours.

Nutrition information: Calories per serving:362; Carbohydrates: 3g; Protein: 23.8g; Fat: 15.3g; Sugar: 0g; Sodium: 724mg; Fiber: 2.4g

Strip Steak with Poblano Peppers

Serves: 4
Preparation time: 3 minutes
Cooking time: 12 hours

Ingredients
- 2 New York strip steaks
- ¼ teaspoon smoked paprika
- 2 poblano peppers, sliced
- 1 onion, cut into wedges
- 1 tablespoon sesame oil

Instructions
1. Place all ingredients except for the sesame oil in the crockpot.
2. Add a few tablespoons of water.
3. Give a good stir.
4. Close the lid and cook on low for 12 hours or on high for 10 hours.
5. Pour sesame oil before serving.

Nutrition information: Calories per serving: 470; Carbohydrates: 2.6g; Protein: 26.3g; Fat: 20.5g; Sugar: 0g; Sodium: 528mg; Fiber: 1.3g

Pan "Grilled" Flank Steak

Serves: 4
Preparation time: 8 minutes
Cooking time: 10 hours

Ingredients

- 1 ½ pounds flank steak, fat trimmed
- Salt and pepper to taste
- A pinch of rosemary
- 1 tablespoon butter, melted
- 1 tablespoon parsley, chopped

Instructions

1. Season the flank steak with salt and pepper to taste.
2. Rub with a pinch of rosemary.
3. Pour the butter in the crockpot and add the slices of flank steak.
4. Close the lid and cook on low for 10 hours or on high for 8 hours.
5. Garnish with parsley before serving.

Nutrition information: Calories per serving: 397; Carbohydrates: 1g; Protein:26.3 g; Fat: 20.7g; Sugar: 0g; Sodium:644mg; Fiber: 0.3g

Baked Sirloin in Crockpot

Serves: 8
Preparation time: 10 minutes
Cooking time: 12 hours

Ingredients

- 2 pounds sirloin steak, cut into 1-inch pieces
- 1 ½ tablespoons cumin
- Salt and pepper to taste
- 2 small red onions, cut into wedges
- 2 red bell peppers, cut into strips

Instructions

1. Season the steak with cumin, salt, and pepper.
2. Grease a skillet and heat over medium flame. Sear the steak for 2 minutes on each side.
3. Add the onions and sear until the edges turn brown.
4. Place into the crockpot.
5. Add a few tablespoons of water.
6. Close the lid and cook on low for 10 hours or on high for 7 hours.
7. An hour before the cooking time ends, stir in the red bell peppers.
8. Cook until the bell peppers become soft.

Nutrition information: Calories per serving: 532; Carbohydrates: 3g; Protein: 34.2g; Fat: 12.6g; Sugar: 0g; Sodium: 613mg; Fiber:1.8 g

Citrus-Rubbed Skirt Steak

Serves: 5
Preparation time: 5 minutes
Cooking time: 12 hours

Ingredients

- 2 teaspoons grated lemon rind
- 2 teaspoons grated orange rind
- Salt and pepper to taste
- 1 clove of garlic, minced
- 1-pound skirt steak

Instructions

1. Line the bottom of the crockpot with foil.
2. In a bowl, mix the lemon rind, orange rind, salt, pepper, and garlic.
3. Rub the spice mix onto the skirt steak.
4. Place inside the crockpot and cook on low for 10 hours or on high for 7 hours.

Nutrition information: Calories per serving: 362; Carbohydrates: 2.3g; Protein: 32.6g; Fat: 15.2g; Sugar: 0g; Sodium: 471mg; Fiber:1.6 g

Flank Steak with Arugula

Serves: 4
Preparation time: 5 minutes
Cooking time: 10 hours

Ingredients

- 1-pound flank steak
- 1 teaspoon Worcestershire sauce
- Salt and pepper to taste
- 1 package arugula salad mix
- 2 tablespoon balsamic vinegar

Instructions

1. Season the flank steak with Worcestershire sauce, salt, and pepper.
2. Place in the crockpot that has been lined with aluminum foil.
3. Close the lid and cook on low for 10 hours or on high for 7 hours.
4. Meanwhile, prepare the salad by combining the arugula salad mix and balsamic vinegar. Set aside in the fridge.
5. Once the steak is cooked, allow to cool before slicing.
6. Serve on top of the arugula salad.

Nutrition information: Calories per serving: 452; Carbohydrates: 5.8g; Protein: 30.2g; Fat:29.5g; Sugar: 1.2g; Sodium: 563mg; Fiber:3 g

Filet Mignon with Fresh Basil Rub

Serves: 4
Preparation time: 5 minutes
Cooking time: 7 hours

Ingredients
- 1 ½ teaspoon fresh basil, minced
- 1 ½ teaspoon thyme, minced
- 4 beef tenderloin steaks, cut to 1-inch thick
- 2 teaspoons garlic, minced
- Salt and pepper to taste

Instructions
1. Line the bottom of the crockpot with foil.
2. In a mixing bowl, combine the basil, thyme, and garlic. Season with salt and pepper.
3. Rub the steaks with the spice rub. Allow to marinate for at least 30 minutes.
4. Place inside the crockpot and cook on high for 7 hours or on low for 10 hours.

Nutrition information: Calories per serving: 424; Carbohydrates: 2.4g; Protein: 30.6g; Fat: 26.3g; Sugar: 0g; Sodium: 537mg; Fiber: 0.8g

Beef-Stuffed Peppers

Serves: 8
Preparation time: 9 minutes
Cooking time:5 hours

Ingredients
- 1-pound lean ground beef
- 1 can tomatoes and chilies
- 1 teaspoon cumin
- 8 medium sweet peppers, top and seeds removed
- 2 cups Mexican cheese blend

Instructions
1. Heat skillet over medium flame and add the ground beef. Stir for 3 minutes until lightly brown.
2. Add the tomatoes and cumin. Turn off the heat and allow to cool.
3. Spoon the beef mixture into the sweet peppers. Top with the Mexican cheese blend.
4. Place inside the crockpot and close the lid.
5. Cook on low for 5 hours or on high for 3 hours.

Nutrition information: Calories per serving: 301; Carbohydrates: 2.5g; Protein:29 g; Fat: 14g; Sugar:0.3 g; Sodium: 797mg; Fiber: 3g

Mexican Bubble Pizza

Serves: 6
Preparation time: 7 minutes
Cooking time: 6 hours

Ingredients
- 1 ½ pound ground beef
- 1 tablespoon taco seasoning
- 2 cups cheddar cheese, shredded
- 1 cup mozzarella cheese
- 1 can condensed tomato soup

Instructions
1. Heat skillet over medium flame and brown the ground beef for a few minutes. Stir in taco seasoning.
2. Place the cheddar cheese into the crockpot.
3. Add the sautéed ground beef on top of the cheddar cheese.
4. Pour the tomato sauce.
5. Sprinkle with mozzarella cheese on top.
6. Close the lid and cook on low for 6 hours and on high for 4 hours.

Nutrition information: Calories per serving: 643; Carbohydrates: 5g; Protein: 45g; Fat: 35g; Sugar:2.1 g; Sodium: 1870mg; Fiber: 2.6g

Barbecue Crockpot Meatloaf

Serves: 6
Preparation time: 5 minutes
Cooking time: 10 hours

Ingredients
- 1-pound ground beef
- 1 cup cheddar cheese
- 2 eggs, beaten
- Salt and pepper to taste
- 2 tablespoon liquid smoke

Instructions
1. Place all ingredients in a mixing bowl.
2. Scoop the mixture into greased ramekins.
3. Place the ramekins inside the crockpot.
4. Pour water into the crockpot such that 1/8 of the ramekins are soaked.
5. Close the lid and cook on low for 10 hours or on high for 7 hours.

Nutrition information: Calories per serving: 330; Carbohydrates:2 g; Protein:21 g; Fat:17 g; Sugar: 0g; Sodium: 668mg; Fiber: 0.7g

CrockPot Beef Stroganoff

Serves: 8
Cook Time: 10 hours

Ingredients

- 2 pounds beef stew meat, sliced into strips
- 2 teaspoons salt
- ½ teaspoon white ground pepper
- 4 cloves of garlic, minced
- 2 teaspoons paprika
- 1 teaspoon thyme
- 1 onion, chopped finely
- 1 cup fresh Portobello mushrooms, sliced
- 1/3 coconut cream
- 2 teaspoon wine vinegar

Instructions

1. Place all ingredients in the CrockPot.
2. Close the lid and cook on high for 8 hours or on low for 10 hours.

Nutrition information: Calories per serving:141; Carbohydrates: 4.2g; Protein:13.2 g; Fat: 8.5g; Sugar: 0g; Sodium: 419mg; Fiber:0.2g

Spicy Beef Curry

Serves: 6
Cook Time: 10 hours

Ingredients

- 2 ½ pounds beef chuck, cubed
- 1 onion, chopped
- 2 tablespoons curry powder
- 3 cloves of garlic, minced
- ½-inch ginger, grated
- 2 cups coconut milk, unsweetened
- Salt and pepper to taste

Instructions

1. Place all ingredients in the CrockPot.
2. Close the lid and cook on high for 8 hours or on low for 10 hours.

Nutrition information: Calories per serving: 455; Carbohydrates:4.5 g; Protein: 41.3g; Fat: 30.2g; Sugar: 0g; Sodium: 729mg; Fiber: 2.6g

CrockPot Beef Stew

Serves: 8
Cook Time: 10 hours

Ingredients

- 1-pound grass-fed beef stew meat, cubed
- 1 onion, chopped
- 1 cup tomatoes, crushed
- 2 cloves of garlic, minced
- 4 sprigs of thyme
- 3 stalks of celery, chopped
- 2 bay leaves
- 2 tablespoons parsley, chopped
- 2 tablespoons apple cider vinegar
- Salt and pepper to taste

Instructions

1. Place all ingredients in the CrockPot.
2. Close the lid and cook on high for 8 hours or on low for 10 hours.

Nutrition information: Calories per serving:124; Carbohydrates: 2.1g; Protein: 11.5g; Fat: 8.9g; Sugar: 0g; Sodium: 420mg; Fiber: 0.8g

Easy CrockPot Roast Beef

Serves: 8
Cook Time: 10 hours

Ingredients

- 1 teaspoon salt
- 1 teaspoon garlic, minced
- ¼ teaspoon rosemary
- ¼ teaspoon thyme
- ¼ teaspoon dried basil
- ¼ teaspoon dried parsley
- ¼ teaspoon dried oregano
- 2 ½ pounds chuck roast, bones removed
- 2 tablespoons olive oil
- 1 cup beef broth
- ¼ cup apple cider vinegar
- ¾ teaspoon salt
- 4 stalks of celery, chopped
- 1 onion, chopped
- 2 bay leaves

Instructions

1. Mix in a small bowl the first 7 ingredients to create the spice rub.
2. Rub the spice mixture onto the beef and allow to marinate for at least 2 hours in the fridge.
3. Place the beef in the CrockPot and add the rest of the ingredients.
4. Close the lid and cook on high for 8 hours or on low for 10 hours.

Nutrition information: Calories per serving: 499; Carbohydrates:3.4 g; Protein: 65.5g; Fat:23.1 g; Sugar: 0.4g; Sodium: 1160mg; Fiber: 1.4g

CrockPot Mexican Beef Stew

Serves: 4
Cook Time: 10 hours

Ingredients

- 1-pound beef stew meat, cubed
- 1 red onion, chopped
- 5 cloves of garlic, minced
- 3 beefsteak tomatoes, chopped
- ¼ cup green chilies, diced
- 1 teaspoon dried oregano
- 1 teaspoon cumin powder
- 2 cups homemade beef broth or water
- Salt and pepper to taste

Instructions

1. Throw all ingredients in the CrockPot.
2. Give a good stir.
3. Close the lid and cook on high for 8 hours or on low for 10 hours.

Nutrition information: Calories per serving:146; Carbohydrates: 3.2g; Protein: 10.4g; Fat: 10.3g; Sugar: 0g; Sodium: 618mg; Fiber: 1.5g

CrockPot Asian Pot Roast

Serves: 6
Cook Time: 10 hours

Ingredients

- 2 pounds beef chuck roast, excess fat trimmed
- 1 ½ teaspoon salt
- 3.4 teaspoon ground black pepper
- 2 tablespoons basil, chopped
- 2 large yellow onions, chopped
- 4 cloves of garlic, minced
- 2 star anise pods
- 2 cups beef stock
- 3 tablespoons sesame seed oil

Instructions

1. Place all ingredients except for the sesame oil in the CrockPot.
2. Close the lid and cook on high for 8 hours or on low for 10 hours.
3. Once cooked, drizzle with sesame seed oil or sesame seeds. You can also garnish it with chopped scallions if desired.

Nutrition information: Calories per serving: 334; Carbohydrates: 2.3g; Protein: 32.3g; Fat: 20.1g; Sugar: 0g; Sodium: 768mg; Fiber: 0.7g

CrockPot Shin Beef

Serves: 2
Cook Time: 10 hours

Ingredients

- 1-pound shin-beef, cut into strips
- 2 tablespoons tallow
- 1 onion, chopped
- 3 stalks of celery, chopped
- 1 cup beef stock
- 1 teaspoon cumin powder
- 1 teaspoon dried thyme
- Salt and pepper to taste

Instructions

1. Place all ingredients in the CrockPot.
2. Give a good stir.
3. Close the lid and cook on high for 8 hours or on low for 10 hours.

Nutrition information: Calories per serving:429; Carbohydrates: 6.3g; Protein: 52.8g; Fat: 20.7g; Sugar: 0g; Sodium: 827mg; Fiber: 3.4g

CrockPot Ground Beef Minestrone Soup

Serves: 4
Cook Time: 8 hours

Ingredients

- 1-pound ground beef
- 2 zucchinis, diced
- 1 onion, diced
- 1 stalk of celery, diced
- ½ cup homemade vegetable broth or water
- 1 clove of garlic, minced
- ½ teaspoon dried basil

Instructions

1. Place all ingredients in the CrockPot.
2. Give a good stir.
3. Close the lid and cook on high for 6 hours or on low for 8 hours.

Nutrition information: Calories per serving: 312; Carbohydrates: 4.8g; Protein: 29.6g; Fat: 18.7g; Sugar: 0.9g; Sodium: 781mg; Fiber: 3.1g

Easy CrockPot Meatballs

Serves: 6
Cook Time: 10 hours

Ingredients

- 2 tablespoons olive oil
- 2 pounds ground beef
- 1 tablespoon cumin
- 1 teaspoon paprika
- 2 eggs, beaten
- 3 cloves of garlic, minced
- 1 tablespoon dried parsley
- Salt and pepper to taste

Instructions

1. Grease the bottom of the CrockPot with olive oil.
2. Place all ingredients in the mixing bowl.
3. Form small balls using your hands and place inside the CrockPot.
4. Close the lid and cook on high for 6 hours or on low for 10 hours.
5. Halfway through the cooking time, turn or flip the meatballs.
6. Close the lid and continue cooking until meat is cooked through.

Nutrition information: Calories per serving: 413; Carbohydrates: 2.5g; Protein: 46.7g; Fat: 21.4g; Sugar: 0g; Sodium: 842mg; Fiber: 0.9g

Spicy Indian Beef Roast

Serves: 8
Cook Time: 10 hours

Ingredients

- 2 red onions, chopped
- 2 tablespoon coconut oil
- 1 teaspoon black mustard seed
- 2 ½ pounds grass-fed beef roast
- 25 curry leaves
- 2 tablespoons lemon juice, freshly squeezed
- 4 cloves of garlic, minced
- 1 ½-inch ginger, minced
- 1 serrano pepper, minced
- 1 tablespoon meat masala

Instructions

1. Place all ingredients in the CrockPot.
2. Give a good stir.
3. Close the lid and cook on high for 6 hours or on low for 10 hours.

Nutrition information: Calories per serving: 222; Carbohydrates: 1.1g; Protein: 31.3g; Fat:10.4 g; Sugar: 0g; Sodium: 544mg; Fiber: 0.5g

CrockPot Beef Picadillo

Serves: 8
Cook Time: 10 hours

Ingredients

- 2 pounds ground beef
- 1 ½ tablespoons chili powder
- 2 tablespoon dried oregano
- 1 teaspoon cinnamon powder
- 1 cup tomatoes, chopped
- 1 red onions, chopped
- 2 Anaheim peppers, seeded and chopped
- 20 green olives, pitted and chopped
- 8 cloves of garlic, minced
- Salt and pepper to taste

Instructions

1. Place all ingredients in the CrockPot.
2. Give a good stir.
3. Close the lid and cook on high for 8 hours or on low for 10 hours.

Nutrition information: Calories per serving: 317; Carbohydrates: 4.5g; Protein: 29.6g; Fat: 19.8g; Sugar: 0g; Sodium: 862mg; Fiber: 2.7g

CrockPot Beef Rendang

Serves: 8
Cook Time: 10 hours

Ingredients

- ½ cup desiccated coconut, toasted
- 6 dried birds eye chilies, chopped
- 1 teaspoon ground cumin
- 2 teaspoon ground coriander
- 1 teaspoon turmeric powder
- 1 teaspoon salt
- 6 cloves of garlic, minced
- ½ cup water
- 1 tablespoon coconut oil
- 6 kafir lime leaves
- 2 stalks lemon grass
- 1 cup coconut cream
- 1 beef shoulder, cut into chunks
- ½ cup cilantro leaves, chopped

Instructions

1. Place all ingredients except the cilantro leaves in the CrockPot.
2. Give a good stir.
3. Close the lid and cook on high for 8 hours or on low for 10 hours.
4. Garnish with cilantro once cooked.

Nutrition information: Calories per serving:305; Carbohydrates: 6.5g; Protein: 32.3g; Fat: 18.7g; Sugar: 0g; Sodium: 830mg; Fiber: 3.7g

Lamb's Feet Soup

Serves: 8
Cook Time: 10 hours

Ingredients

- 1 ½ pounds lamb's feet
- 1 onion, chopped
- 1 cup tomatoes, crushed
- 1 teaspoon coriander seeds
- 1 teaspoon black peppercorns
- 1-inch ginger, grated
- 3 cloves of garlic, minced
- 1 bay leaf
- 4 cups water

Instructions

1. Place all ingredients in the CrockPot.
2. Give a good stir.
3. Close the lid and cook on high for 8 hours or on low for 10 hours.

Nutrition information: Calories per serving: 229; Carbohydrates: 2.4g; Protein: 21.6g; Fat:14.9 g; Sugar: 0g; Sodium: 528mg; Fiber: 1.7g

Onion and Bison Soup

Serves: 8
Cook Time: 10 hours

Ingredients

- 6 onions, julienned
- 2 pounds bison meat, cubed
- 3 cups beef stock
- ½ cup sherry
- 3 sprigs of thyme
- 1 bay leaf
- 2 tablespoons olive oil
- Salt and pepper to taste

Instructions

1. Place all ingredients in the CrockPot.
2. Give a good stir.
3. Close the lid and cook on high for 8 hours or on low for 10 hours.

Nutrition information: Calories per serving: 341; Carbohydrates: 9.5g; Protein: 24.5g; Fat: 21.8g; Sugar: 1.7g; Sodium: 809mg; Fiber: 4.8g

CrockPot Moroccan Beef

Serves: 8
Cook Time: 10 hours

Ingredients

- 2 pounds beef roast, cut into strips
- ½ cup onions, sliced
- 4 tablespoons garam masala
- 1 teaspoon salt
- ½ cup bone broth

Instructions

1. Place all ingredients in the CrockPot.
2. Give a good stir.
3. Close the lid and cook on high for 8 hours or on low for 10 hours.

Nutrition information: Calories per serving: 310; Carbohydrates: 0.7g; Protein: 30.3g; Fat: 25.5g; Sugar: 0g; Sodium: 682mg; Fiber: 0.5g

CrockPot Creamy Beef Bourguignon

Serves: 8
Cook Time: 10 hours

Ingredients

- 3 beef steaks, cut into large chunks
- 3 tablespoons lard
- 3 cloves of garlic, minced
- 1 onion, diced
- 1 tablespoon organic tomato puree
- 4 cups white mushrooms, sliced
- 1 cup homemade chicken stock
- Salt and pepper to taste
- ½ cup heavy cream

Instructions

1. Place all ingredients except the cream in the CrockPot.
2. Give a good stir.
3. Close the lid and cook on high for 8 hours or on low for 10 hours.

Nutrition information: Calories per serving: 678; Carbohydrates: 4.3g; Protein: 36.7g; Fat: 45g; Sugar: 0g; Sodium: 826mg; Fiber:1.3g

Lamb with Mint

Serves: 4
Cook Time: 10 hours

Ingredients

- 2 tablespoons ghee
- 1 lamb leg, bone in
- 4 cloves of garlic, minced
- ¼ cup fresh mint, chopped
- ½ teaspoon salt
- A dash of ground black pepper

Instructions

1. Heat oil in skillet over medium flame.
2. Sear the lamb leg for at least 3 minutes on each side.
3. Place in the CrockPot and add the rest of the ingredients.
4. Close the lid and cook on high for 8 hours or on low for 8 hours.

Nutrition information: Calories per serving: 525; Carbohydrates: 6.5g; Protein: 37.4g; Fat: 18.3g; Sugar:0g; Sodium: 748mg; Fiber: 2.4g

CrockPot Lamb Roast

Serves: 8
Cook Time: 8 hours

Ingredients

- 2 pounds leg of lamb
- ¼ cup olive oil
- 2 tablespoons mustard
- 4 sprigs thyme
- 7 leaves of mint
- ¾ teaspoon dried rosemary
- 4 cloves of garlic
- Salt and pepper to taste

Instructions

1. Mix all ingredients in the mixing bowl. Allow to rest in the fridge to marinate.
2. Line the bottom of the CrockPot with aluminum foil.
3. Grease the foil with butter or ghee.
4. Place the lamb leg in the CrockPot.
5. Close the lid and cook on high for 8 hours or on low for 10 hours.

Nutrition information: Calories per serving: 414; Carbohydrates: 0.3g; Protein: 26.7g; Fat: 35.2g; Sugar: 0g; Sodium: 827mg; Fiber: 0g

Lamb with Thyme

Serves: 2
Cook Time: 10 hours

Ingredients

- 2 lamb shoulder chops, bone in
- 1 cup homemade chicken broth
- 1 teaspoon garlic paste
- ¼ cup thyme sprigs, chopped
- Salt and pepper to taste

Instructions

1. Place all ingredients in the CrockPot.
2. Give a good stir.
3. Close the lid and cook on high for 8 hours or on low for 10 hours.

Nutrition information: Calories per serving: 767; Carbohydrates: 4.3g; Protein: 95.4g; Fat: 41.5g; Sugar: 0g; Sodium: 1147mg; Fiber: 3.2g

CrockPot Lamb Chops

Serves: 6
Cook Time: 10 hours

Ingredients

- 6 lamb shanks
- 1 tablespoon olive oil
- 2 teaspoons salt
- 2 teaspoons pepper
- 2 stalks of celery, chopped
- 1 onion, chopped
- 1 tablespoon dried oregano
- 1 ½ cups chicken stock
- 1 cup tomatoes, crushed
- 3 bay leaves

Instructions

1. Place all ingredients in the CrockPot.
2. Give a good stir.
3. Close the lid and cook on high for 8 hours or on low for 10 hours.

Nutrition information: Calories per serving: 762; Carbohydrates: 3.2g; Protein: 98g; Fat: 31g; Sugar: 0g; Sodium: 1816mg; Fiber: 2.1g

Spicy Eggplant with Red Pepper and Parsley

Serves: 4
Preparation time: 3 minutes
Cooking time: 3 hours

Ingredients
- 1 large eggplant, sliced
- 2 tablespoons parsley, chopped
- 1 big red bell pepper, chopped
- Salt and pepper to taste
- 2 tablespoons balsamic vinegar

Instructions
1. Place all ingredients in a mixing bowl.
2. Toss to coat ingredients.
3. Place in the crockpot and cook on low for 3 hours or on high for 1 hour.

Nutrition information: Calories per serving: 52; Carbohydrates:11.67 g; Protein:1.8 g; Fat:0.31 g; Sugar: 0.2g; Sodium: 142mg; Fiber: 9.4g

Spinach with Halloumi Cheese Casserole

Serves: 4
Preparation time: 5 minutes
Cooking time: 2 hours

Ingredients
- 1 package spinach, rinsed
- ½ cup walnuts, chopped
- Salt and pepper to taste
- 1 tablespoon balsamic vinegar
- 1 ½ cups halloumi cheese, grated

Instructions
1. Place spinach and walnuts in the crockpot.
2. Season with salt and pepper. Drizzle with balsamic vinegar.
3. Top with halloumi cheese and cook on low for 2 hours or on high for 30 minutes

Nutrition information: Calories per serving: 560; Carbohydrates: 7g; Protein:21 g; Fat: 47g; Sugar:2.1 g; Sodium: 231mg; Fiber:3 g

Crockpot Baked Tofu

Serves: 4
Preparation time: 2 hours 5 minutes
Cooking time: 2 hours

Ingredients

- 1 small package extra firm tofu, sliced
- 3 tablespoons soy sauce
- 1 tablespoon sesame oil
- 2 teaspoons minced garlic
- Juice from ½ lemon, freshly squeezed

Instructions

1. In a deep dish, mix together the soy sauce, sesame oil, garlic, and lemon. Add a few tablespoons of water if the sauce is too thick.
2. Marinate the tofu slices for at least 2 hours.
3. Line the crockpot with foil and grease it with cooking spray.
4. Place the slices of marinated tofu into the crockpot.
5. Cook on low for 4 hours or on high for 2 hours.
6. Make sure that the tofu slices have a crispy outer texture.

Nutrition information: Calories per serving:145; Carbohydrates: 4.1g; Protein: 11.6g; Fat: 10.8g; Sugar: 0.6g; Sodium: 142mg; Fiber:1.5 g

Cream of Mushroom Soup

Serves: 4
Preparation time: 6 minutes
Cooking time: 3 hours

Ingredients

- 1 tablespoons olive oil
- ½ cup onion, diced
- 20 ounces mushrooms, sliced
- 2 cups chicken broth
- 1 cup heavy cream

Instructions

1. In a skillet, heat the oil over medium flame and sauté the onions until translucent or slightly brown on the edges.
2. Transfer into the crockpot and add the mushrooms and chicken broth. Season with salt and pepper to taste.
3. Close the lid and cook on low for 6 hours or on high for 3 hours until the mushrooms are soft
4. Halfway before the cooking time ends, stir in the heavy cream.

Nutrition information: Calories per serving: 229; Carbohydrates: 9g; Protein: 5g; Fat: 21g; Sugar:3 g; Sodium:214 mg; Fiber: 2g

Broccoli and Cheese Casserole

Serves: 4
Preparation time: 5 minutes
Cooking time: 4 hours

Ingredients
- ¾ cup almond flour
- 1 head of broccoli, cut into florets
- 2 large eggs, beaten
- Salt and pepper to taste
- ½ cup mozzarella cheese

Instructions
1. Place the almond flour and broccoli in the crockpot.
2. Stir in the eggs and season with salt and pepper to taste.
3. Sprinkle with mozzarella cheese.
4. Close the lid and cook on low for 4 hours or on high for 2 hours.

Nutrition information: Calories per serving: 78; Carbohydrates: 4g; Protein: 8.2g; Fat:5.8 g; Sugar: 0g; Sodium: 231mg; Fiber:2.3 g

Asian Broccoli Sauté

Serves: 4
Preparation time: 3 minutes
Cooking time: 3 hours

Ingredients
- 1 tablespoon coconut oil
- 1 head broccoli, cut into florets
- 1 tablespoon coconut aminos or soy sauce
- 1 teaspoon ginger, grated
- Salt and pepper to taste

Instructions
1. Place the ingredients in the crockpot.
2. Toss everything to combine.
3. Close the lid and cook on low for 3 hours or on high for an hour.
4. Once cooked, sprinkle with sesame seeds or sesame oil.

Nutrition information: Calories per serving: 62; Carbohydrates:3.6 g; Protein: 1.8g; Fat: 4.3g; Sugar:0.3 g; Sodium: 87mg; Fiber: 2.1g

Vegetarian Red Coconut Curry

Serves: 4
Preparation time: 3 minutes
Cooking time: 3 hours

Ingredients
- 1 cup broccoli florets
- 1 large handful spinach, rinsed
- 1 tablespoon red curry paste
- 1 cup coconut cream
- 1 teaspoon garlic, minced

Instructions
1. Combine all ingredients in the crockpot.
2. Close the lid and cook on low for 3 hours or on high for 1 hour.

Nutrition information: Calories per serving: 226; Carbohydrates: 8g; Protein: 5.2g; Fat:21.4 g; Sugar: 0.4g; Sodium: 341mg; Fiber:4.3 g

Eggplant Parmesan Casserole

Serves: 3
Preparation time: 5 minutes
Cooking time: 3 hours

Ingredients
- 1 medium eggplant, sliced
- 1 large egg
- Salt and pepper to taste
- 1 cup almond flour
- 1 cup parmesan cheese

Instructions
1. Place the eggplant slices in the crockpot.
2. Pour in the eggs and season with salt and pepper.
3. Stir in the almond flour and sprinkle with parmesan cheese.
4. Stir to combine everything.
5. Close the lid and cook on low for 3 hours or on high for 2 hours.

Nutrition information: Calories per serving: 212; Carbohydrates: 17g; Protein: 15g; Fat:12.1 g; Sugar: 1.2g; Sodium: 231mg; Fiber:8.1 g

Vegetarian Keto Burgers

Serves: 4
Preparation time: 8 minutes
Cooking time: 4 hours

Ingredients
- 2 Portobello mushrooms, chopped
- 2 tablespoons basil, chopped
- 1 clove of garlic, minced
- 1 egg, beaten
- ½ cup boiled cauliflower, mashed

Instructions
1. Line the bottom of the crockpot with foil.
2. In a food processor, combine all ingredients.
3. Make 4 burger patties using your hands and place gently in the crockpot.
4. Close the lid and cook on low for 4 hours or on high for 3 hours.

Nutrition information: Calories per serving: 134; Carbohydrates: 18g; Protein: 10g; Fat: 3.1g; Sugar:0.9g; Sodium:235mg; Fiber: 5g

Garlic Gnocchi

Serves: 4
Preparation time: 15 minutes
Cooking time: 3 hours

Ingredients
- 2 cups mozzarella, shredded
- 3 egg yolks, beaten
- 1 teaspoon garlic, minced
- ½ cup heavy cream
- Salt and pepper to taste

Instructions
1. In a mixing bowl, combine the mozzarella and egg yolks.
2. Form gnocchi balls and place in the fridge to set.
3. Boil a pot of water over high flame and drop the gnocchi balls for 30 seconds. Take them out and transfer to the crockpot.
4. Into the crockpot add the garlic and heavy cream.
5. Season with salt and pepper to taste.
6. Close the lid and cook on low for 3 hours or on high for 1 hour.

Nutrition information: Calories per serving: 178; Carbohydrates: 4.1g; Protein:20.5 g; Fat: 8.9g; Sugar:0.3g; Sodium: 421mg; Fiber: 2.1g

Lazy Minestrone Soup

Serves: 4
Preparation time: 3 minutes
Cooking time: 3 hours

Ingredients
- 1 cup zucchini, sliced
- 2 cups chicken broth
- 1 package diced vegetables of your choice
- 2 tablespoons basil, chopped
- ½ cup diced celery

Instructions
1. Place all ingredients in the crockpot.
2. Season with salt and pepper to taste.
3. Close the lid and cook on low for 3 hours or on high for 1 hour.

Nutrition information: Calories per serving: 259; Carbohydrates: 13.5g; Protein:30.3 g; Fat: 8.3g; Sugar: 0.4g; Sodium: 643mg; Fiber: 4.2g

Zucchini Basil Soup

Serves: 8
Cook Time: 3 hours

Ingredients
- 9 cups zucchini, diced
- 2 cups white onions, chopped
- 4 cups vegetable broth
- 8 cloves of garlic, minced
- 1 cup basil leaves
- 4 tablespoons olive oil
- Salt and pepper to taste

Instructions
1. Place the ingredients in the CrockPot.
2. Give a good stir.
3. Close the lid and cook on high for 2 hours or on low for 3 hours.
4. Once cooked, transfer into a blender and pulse until smooth.

Nutrition information: Calories per serving: 93; Carbohydrates: 5.4g; Protein: 1.3g; Fat: 11.6g; Sugar: 0g; Sodium: 322mg; Fiber: 4.2g

CrockPot Cumin-Roasted Vegetables

Serves: 2

Ingredients

- 1 red bell pepper, chopped
- 1 yellow bell pepper, chopped
- 1 green bell pepper, chopped
- ½ cup cherry tomatoes
- ¼ cup pepita seeds
- 6 cups kale leaves, chopped
- 4 tablespoon olive oil
- 1 teaspoon cumin
- 1 teaspoon dried oregano
- ¼ teaspoon salt

Instructions

1. Place all ingredients in a mixing bowl. Toss to coat everything with oil.
2. Line the bottom of the CrockPot with foil.
3. Place the vegetables inside.
4. Close the lid and cook on low for 4 hours or on high for 6 hours until the vegetables are a bit brown on the edges.

Nutrition information: Calories per serving:380; Carbohydrates: 13.8g; Protein: 8.6g; Fat:35.8g; Sugar:1.7 g; Sodium: 512mg; Fiber: 6.6g

CrockPot Eggplant Lasagna

Serves: 4
Cook Time: 4 hours

Ingredients

- 1 cup beefsteak tomatoes
- ½ cup basil leaves
- ½ teaspoon thyme leaves
- 1 onion, diced
- 1 red bell pepper diced
- Salt and pepper to taste
- 1 cup chopped walnuts
- 2 large eggs, beaten
- 1 cup heavy cream
- 2 tablespoons olive oil
- 1 eggplant, sliced using a mandolin
- 1 cup mozzarella cheese

Instructions

1. In a blender or food processor, combine the tomatoes, basil leaves, thyme leaves, onion, and red bell pepper. Season with salt and pepper then pulse until smooth. Place in a bowl and add the chopped walnuts.
2. In another bowl, combine the eggs and heavy cream. Set aside.
3. Grease the bottom of the CrockPot with olive oil.
4. Arrange the eggplant slices first and pour in a generous amount of the tomato sauce mixture. Pour the egg mixture and cheese on top.
5. Repeat the layering until all ingredients are used up.
6. Close the lid and cook on high for 3 hours or on low for 4 hours.

Nutrition information: Calories per serving: 373; Carbohydrates: 19g; Protein: 23g; Fat: 14g; Sugar: 1.2g; Sodium: 963mg; Fiber: 13.8g

Cauliflower Mac and Cheese

Serves: 6
Cook Time: 4 hours

Ingredients

- 1 large cauliflower, cut into small florets
- 2 tablespoons butter
- 1 cup heavy cream
- 2 ounces grass-fed cream cheese
- 1 ½ teaspoons Dijon mustard
- 1 ½ cup organic sharp cheddar cheese
- 1 tablespoon garlic powder
- ½ cup nutritional yeast
- Salt and pepper to taste

Instructions

1. Place all ingredients in the CrockPot.
2. Give a good stir.
3. Close the lid and cook on high for 3 hours or on low for 4 hours.

Nutrition information: Calories per serving:329; Carbohydrates: 10.8g; Protein: 16.1g; Fat: 25.5g; Sugar: 0g; Sodium: 824mg; Fiber: 5.8g

Baby Kale, Mozzarella and Egg Bake

Serves: 6
Cook Time: 4 hours

Ingredients

- 2 cups baby kale, chopped
- 2 teaspoons olive oil
- 1 ½ cup mozzarella cheese, grated
- 8 eggs, beaten
- 1 teaspoon garlic powder
- 1 teaspoon onion powder
- Salt and pepper to taste

Instructions

1. Place all ingredients in the CrockPot.
2. Give a good stir.
3. Close the lid and cook on high for 3 hours or on low for 4 hours.

Nutrition information: Calories per serving: 352; Carbohydrates:6.3 g; Protein: 32.1g; Fat: 21.6g; Sugar: 0.9g; Sodium: 841mg; Fiber: 3.7g

Zucchini Soup with Rosemary and Parmesan

Serves: 6
Cook Time: 3 hours

Ingredients

- 2 tablespoons olive oil
- 1 tablespoon butter
- 1 onion, chopped
- 1 teaspoon minced garlic
- 1 teaspoon Italian seasoning
- 4 teaspoons rosemary, chopped
- 2 pounds zucchini, chopped
- 8 cups vegetable stock
- Salt and pepper to taste
- 1 cup grated parmesan cheese

Instructions

1. Place all ingredients except for the parmesan cheese in the CrockPot.
2. Give a good stir.
3. Close the lid and cook on high for 3 hours or on low for 4 hours
4. Place inside a blender and pulse until smooth.
5. Serve with parmesan cheese on top.

Nutrition information: Calories per serving: 172; Carbohydrates: 5.9g; Protein: 9.2g; Fat: 13.7g; Sugar: 0g; Sodium: 367mg; Fiber: 2.6g

Creamy Keto Mash

Serves: 3
Cook Time: 4 hours

Ingredients

- 1 cauliflower head, cut into florets
- 1 white onion, chopped
- 2 cloves of garlic, minced
- ¼ cup vegetable stock
- ¼ cup butter
- Salt and pepper to taste
- ½ cup cream cheese

Instructions

1. Place the all ingredients except for the cream cheese in the CrockPot.
2. Close the lid and cook on high for 3 hours or on low for 4 hours.
3. Place in the food processor and pour in the cream cheese. Pulse until slightly fine.
4. Garnish with chopped parsley if desired.

Nutrition information: Calories per serving: 302; Carbohydrates: 7g; Protein: 3.7g; Fat: 28g; Sugar: 0g; Sodium: 771mg; Fiber: 3.8g

CrockPot Mediterranean Eggplant Salad

Serves: 2
Cook Time: 4 hours

Ingredients

- 1 red onion, sliced
- 2 bell peppers, sliced
- 3 extra virgin olive oil
- 1 eggplant, quartered
- 1 cup tomatoes, crushed
- 1 tablespoon smoked paprika
- 2 teaspoons cumin
- Juice from 1 lemon, freshly squeezed
- Salt and pepper to taste

Instructions

1. Place all ingredients in the CrockPot.
2. Give a good stir.
3. Close the lid and cook on high for 3 hours or on low for 4 hours.

Nutrition information: Calories per serving: 312; Carbohydrates: 30.2g; Protein: 5.6g; Fat: 22g; Sugar: 0.4g; Sodium: 519mg; Fiber: 27.1g

Curried Vegetable Stew

Serves: 10
Cook Time: 3 hours

Ingredients

- 1 teaspoon olive oil
- 1 onion, diced
- 2 tablespoon curry powder
- 1 tablespoon grated ginger
- 3 cloves of garlic, minced
- 1/8 teaspoon cayenne pepper
- 1 cup tomatoes, crushed
- 1 bag baby spinach
- 1 yellow bell pepper, chopped
- 1 red bell pepper, chopped
- 2 cups vegetable broth
- 1 cup coconut milk
- Salt and pepper to taste

Instructions

1. Place all ingredients in the CrockPot.
2. Give a good stir.
3. Close the lid and cook on high for 2 hours or on low for 3 hours.

Nutrition information: Calories per serving: 88; Carbohydrates: 5.1g; Protein: 2.9g; Fat: 9.3g; Sugar: 0g; Sodium: 318mg; Fiber: 3.9g

CrockPot Vindaloo Vegetables

Serves: 6
Cook Time: 4 hours

Ingredients

- 3 cloves of garlic, minced
- 1 tablespoon ginger, chopped
- 1 ½ teaspoon coriander powder
- 1 ¼ teaspoon ground cumin
- ½ teaspoon dry mustard
- ½ teaspoon cayenne pepper
- ½ teaspoon cardamom
- ½ teaspoon turmeric powder
- 1 onion, chopped
- 4 cups cauliflower florets
- 1 red bell peppers, chopped
- 1 green bell peppers, chopped
- Salt and pepper to taste

Instructions

1. Place all ingredients in the CrockPot.
2. Give a good stir.
3. Close the lid and cook on high for 3 hours or on low for 4 hours.

Nutrition information: Calories per serving: 159; Carbohydrates: 32.6g; Protein: 9g; Fat: 1g; Sugar:0.3g; Sodium: 464mg; Fiber: 25.3g

Herbed Chicken & Green Chiles Soup

Total Cooking Time: 6 hours

Servings: 8 (13.1 ounces per serving)

- 2 chicken breasts, boneless, skinless
- ½ teaspoon cumin, ground
- 1 teaspoon onion powder
- 1 teaspoon chili powder
- 1 teaspoon garlic powder
- ½ teaspoon white pepper, ground
- ¼ teaspoon cayenne pepper
- 4 ounces green chilies
- 1 cup beans
- 3 cups water
- ½ avocado, cubed
- 2 tablespoons extra virgin olive oil
- 1 small carrot, diced

Directions:

Grease the bottom of Crock-Pot with olive oil and place chicken inside pot. Mix white pepper, cumin, garlic, onion, and chili powder. Sprinkle evenly over the chicken. Place the chilies on top of chicken. Pour in water and add beans and carrot and stir. Close the lid and cook on HIGH for an hour. Open the lid and give a good stir. Close the lid and continue to cook on HIGH for 5 hours. Serve hot with avocado.

Nutrition Values:

Calories: 180.02, Total Fat: 7.04 g, Saturated Fat: 1.19 g, Cholesterol: 18.28 mg, Sodium: 831.99 mg, Potassium: 599.6 mg, Total Carbohydrates: 9.82 g, Fiber: 3.93 g, Sugar: 1.6 g, Protein: 13.02 g

Peas & Mushroom Soup (Crock-Pot)

Total Cooking Time: 7 hours and 5 minutes

Servings: 4 (13.5 ounces)

Ingredients:

- 3 cups Cremini mushrooms, thinly sliced
- 1 cup peas, fresh or frozen
- 4 garlic cloves, minced
- 2 tablespoons ginger, fresh, grated
- 4 cups water
- 2 tablespoons tamari (or soy sauce)
- 2 tablespoons wine vinegar
- 1 teaspoon chili paste
- 2 teaspoons sesame oil
- Salt and black pepper, to taste
- Parmesan cheese, freshly grated

Directions:

Place all the ingredients in Crock-Pot. Cover and cook on LOW for 7 hours or on HIGH for 4 hours. When ready sprinkle with grated cheese. Serve hot.

Nutrition Values:

Calories: 215.83 , Total Fat: 3.11 g, Saturated Fat: 0.44 g, Cholesterol: 0 mg, Sodium:

286.92 mg, Potassium: 806.92 mg, Total Carbohydrates: 18 g, Fiber: 13.47 g, Sugar:

2.58 g, Protein: 14.97 g

Minced Beef & Vegetable Soup

Total Cooking Time: 8 hours and 15 minutes

Servings: 6 (8.2 ounces per serving)

Ingredients:

- 1 ½ lbs. lean minced meat (beef)
- 1 sweet potato, cubed
- 2 sticks of celery, sliced
- 3 carrots, sliced
- 2 green onions, finely sliced
- 4 tablespoons tomato paste, sugar-free and low sodium
- 1 ½ cups water
- Salt and black pepper to taste
- ½ cup green beans, chopped

Directions:

In a large skillet, sauté the minced meat over medium-high heat. Drain the fat and set aside. Layer the bottom of Crock-Pot with potatoes. Spread the celery and green beans on top of potatoes, then spread a layer of meat on top of celery. Season with salt and pepper. Add chopped carrots and onions. In a bowl, mix tomato paste and water and pour into Crock Pot over remaining ingredients. Cover and cook for 6-8 hours. Serve hot.

Nutritional Values:

Calories: 323.8, Total Fat: 25.12 g, Saturated Fat: 9.42 g, Cholesterol: 64.86 mg, Sodium: 107.4 mg, Potassium: 586.28 mg, Total Carbohydrates: 8.05 g, Fiber: 2.17 g, Sugar: 3.29 g, Protein: 13.35 g

Sweet Potato & Sausage Soup

Total Cooking Time: 7 hours and 35 minutes

Servings: 6 (12.4 ounces per serving)

Ingredients:

- 1 lb. sausage links, pork or chicken
- 8 large sweet potatoes, cubed
- 1 onion, chopped
- 1 glass red wine
- 4 tablespoons tomato sauce
- Olive oil
- 3 cups water
- Salt and pepper to taste and other seasonings
- 1 cup of bacon, cooked, cubed
- 1 cup smoked ham, cooked, cubed
- 1 red pepper, diced

Directions:

Chop the onion into cubes. Grease a frying pan and sauté onion until golden in color, for about six minutes. Add the cubed ham and bacon. Add cubed potatoes and salt and pepper to taste. Pour in wine and stir. Place all ingredients in Crock Pot. Add the water and cover and cook on LOW for 6-7 hours. Add the chopped pepper and tomato sauce and cook on LOW for an additional 30 minutes more. Serve hot.

Nutritional Values:

Calories: 126.71, Total Fat: 2.02 g, Saturated Fat: 0.99 g, Cholesterol: 18.33 mg, Sodium: 787.22 mg, Potassium: 215.12 mg, Total Carbohydrates: 6.95 g, Fiber: 0.52 g, Sugar: 1.26 g, Protein: 15.3 g

Vegan Cream of Tomato Soup

Total Cooking Time: *3 hours*

Servings: 4

Ingredients:

- 4 Roma tomatoes
- ½ cup sun dried tomatoes
- 1 teaspoon sea salt
- ¼ teaspoon black pepper
- ¼ teaspoon white pepper
- ¼ cup basil, fresh, chopped
- 1 clove of garlic
- 4 cups water

Directions:

Add ingredients to a high-powered blender and blend until smooth, for about 5 minutes. Add the blended mix to Crock-Pot, cook on LOW for 3 hours. Serve hot.

Nutritional Values:

Calories: 187, Total Fat: 15.9 g, Saturated Fat: 2.5 g, Sodium: 538 mg, Carbs: 11.8 g, Dietary Fiber: 4.1 g, Net Carbs: 7.7 g, Sugars: 3.4 g, Protein: 3.5 g

Cream of Broccoli Soup

Total Cooking Time: 3 hours

Servings: 4

Ingredients:

- 1 yellow onion, sliced
- 1 teaspoon extra-virgin olive oil
- 1 teaspoon sea salt
- Fresh ground pepper to taste
- 4 cups cauliflower florets
- 3 cups unsweetened almond milk
- 3 cups broccoli florets, finely chopped
- 1 tablespoon onion powder

Directions:

Sauté the onion in oil in large pan along with salt and pepper over medium-high heat for 5 minutes, adding a few tablespoons of water to pan to avoid burning. Add cauliflower and milk, cover and bring to boil. Reduce heat to simmer and cook, covered, for 10 minutes or until the florets are soft. Add in half the broccoli. Pour mixture into blender or food processor. Puree until smooth. Add mix to Crock-Pot and add remaining broccoli and onion powder. Cover and cook on LOW for 3 hours. Serve hot.

Nutritional Values:

Calories: 123, Total Fat: 3.9 g, Sodium: 678 mg, Carbs: 19 g, Dietary Fiber: 7.5 g, Net Carbs: 11.5 g, Sugars: 7 g, Protein: 6.5 g

Vegan Grain-free Cream of Mushroom Soup

Total Cooking Time: **4 hours**

Servings: 2

Ingredients:

- 2 cups cauliflower florets
- 1 teaspoon onion powder
- 1 2/3 cups unsweetened almond milk
- 1 ½ cups white mushrooms, diced
- ¼ teaspoon Himalayan rock salt
- ½ yellow onion, diced

Directions:

Place onion powder, milk, cauliflower, salt, and pepper in a pan, cover and bring to a boil over medium heat. Reduce heat to low and simmer for 8 minutes or until cauliflower is softened. Then, puree mixture in food processor. In a pan, add oil, mushrooms, and onions, heat over high heat for about 8 minutes. Add mushrooms and onion mix to cauliflower mixture in Crock-Pot. Cover and cook on LOW for 4 hours. Serve hot.

Nutritional Values:

Calories: 95, Total Fat: 4 g, Sodium: 475 mg, Carbs: 12.3 g, Dietary Fiber: 4.4 g, Net Carbs: 7.9 g, Sugars: 4.9 g, Protein: 4.9 g

Roasted Garlic Soup

Total Cooking Time: 3 ½ hours

Servings: 6

Ingredients:

- 1 tablespoon extra-virgin olive oil
- 2 bulbs of garlic
- 3 shallots, chopped
- 6 cups gluten-free vegetable broth
- 1 large head of cauliflower, chopped, about 5 cups
- Fresh ground pepper to taste
- Sea salt to taste

Directions:

Preheat oven to 400° Fahrenheit. Peel the outer layers off garlic bulbs. Cut about 1/4 inch off the top of the bulbs, place into foil pan. Coat bulbs with olive oil, and cook in oven for 35 minutes. Once cooked, allow them to cool. Squeeze the garlic out of the bulbs into your food processor. Meanwhile, in a pan, sauté remaining olive oil and chopped shallots over medium-high heat for about 6 minutes. Add other ingredients to saucepan, cover and reduce heat to a simmer for 20 minutes or until the cauliflower is softened. Add the mixture to food processor and puree until smooth. Add mix to Crock Pot, cover with lid, and cook on LOW for 3 ½ hours. Serve hot.

Nutritional Values:

Calories: 73, Total Fat: 2.4 g, Sodium: 1201 mg, Carbs: 11.3 g, Dietary Fiber: 2.1 g, Net Carbs: 2.1 g, Sugars: 4.1 g, Protein: 2.1 g

Hamburger Soup

Total Cooking Time: **5 hours 45 minutes**

Servings: **6**

Ingredients:

- ½ red onion, sliced
- 10 mushrooms, chopped
- 20 Brussels sprouts, halved
- ¼ cup red palm oil, melted
- Himalayan rock salt, to taste
- 1 yellow bell pepper, sliced
- 1 lb. grass-fed, regular ground beef
- 3 cloves garlic, minced
- 6 sticks of celery, chopped
- 4 cups homemade beef stock, with fat
- 2 cups organic whole tomatoes, chopped
- 1 tablespoon organic tomato paste
- 1 bay leaf
- 1 teaspoon oregano, dried
- Pinch of cayenne pepper
- ¼ cup parsley, fresh, chopped

Directions:

In a pan, brown ground beef over medium-high heat for about 10 minutes. Place bell pepper, mushrooms, brussels sprouts, onions, cover with palm oil and salt and pepper. In the oven, roast veggies for 30 minutes at 350°Fahrenheit. In Crock Pot, add browned beef, celery, garlic. Add in remaining ingredients, cover and cook for 5 hours on LOW. Stir in the roasted vegetables and chopped parsley. Serve hot.

Nutritional Values:

Calories: 478, Total Fat: 34.5 g, Saturated Fat: 14.7 g, Cholesterol: 76 mg, Sodium: 520 mg, Carbs: 13.9 g, Dietary Fiber: 3.2 g, Net Carbs: 10.7 g, Sugars: 4.5 g, Protein: 28.8 g

Crock-Pot Buffalo Chicken Soup

Total Cooking Time: 6 hours

Servings: 5

Ingredients:

- 3 medium chicken thighs, deboned, sliced
- 1 teaspoon garlic powder
- 1 teaspoon onion powder
- ½ teaspoon celery seed
- ¼ cup butter
- ½ cup Frank's hot sauce or to taste, depending on how hot you like it
- 3 cups beef broth
- 1 cup heavy cream
- 2 ounces cream cheese
- ¼ teaspoon Xanthan gum
- Salt and pepper to taste

Directions:

Cut up chicken into chunks and place in Crock-Pot. Add all the other ingredients except the cream cheese and Xanthan gum. Set to Crock-Pot on LOW for 6 hours and allow to cook completely. Once cooking is done, remove the chicken from pot and shred with fork. Add the cream cheese and Xanthan gum to Crock-Pot. Using an immersion blender, emulsify all the liquids together. Add chicken back to Crock-Pot and stir. Season with salt and pepper to taste. Serve hot.

Nutritional Values:Calories: 523.2, Total Fats: 44.2 g, Carbs: 3.4 g, Fiber: 0 g, Net Carbs: 3.4 g, Protein: 20.8 g

Crock-Pot Clam Chowder

Total Cooking Time: 6 hours

Servings: 8

Ingredients:

- 1 cup chopped onion
- 13 slices thick cut bacon
- 1 cup celery, chopped
- 2 cups chicken broth
- 2 cups heavy whipping cream
- 1 teaspoon thyme, ground
- 1 teaspoon sea salt
- 1 teaspoon pepper

Directions:

Cook the bacon until crispy and reserve the bacon grease in pan. Chop celery and onion. Place celery and onion in bacon grease and cook until soft; add grease to Crock-Pot along with veggies. Once veggies are soft, add them to the Crock-Pot and all other ingredients. Cover and cook on LOW for 6 hours.

Nutritional Values:

Calories: 427, Total Fat: 33 g, Cholesterol: 252 mg, Sodium: 1636 mg, Potassium: 107 mg, Carbohydrates: 5 g, Dietary Fiber: 0 g, Sugars: 0 g, Protein: 27 g

Crock-Pot Low-Carb Taco Soup

Total Cooking Time: 4 hours

Servings: 8

Ingredients:

- 2 lbs. ground pork, beef or sausage
- 2 8-ounce packages of cream cheese
- 2 10-ounce cans of Rotel
- 2 tablespoons of taco seasoning
- 4 cups chicken broth
- 2 tablespoons cilantro, fresh or dried
- 1 can corn kernels, drained
- ½ cup cheddar cheese, shredded for garnish (optional)

Directions:

Brown the ground meat until fully cooked over medium-high heat in a pan. While the meat is browning, place cream cheese, Rotel, corn and taco seasoning in Crock-Pot. Drain grease off meat and place meat in Crock-Pot. Stir and combine. Pour chicken broth over mixture, cover and cook on LOW for 4 hours. Just before serving, add in cilantro and garnish with shredded cheddar cheese.

Nutritional Values:

Calories: 547, Total Fat: 43 g, Saturated Fat: 20 g, Carbohydrates: 5 g, Sugar: 4 g

Sodium: 1174 mg, Fiber: 1 g, Cholesterol: 168 mg, Protein: 33 g

Chicken Bacon Orzo Soup

Total Cooking Time: 5 hours

Servings: 6 (1.7 ounces per serving)

Ingredients:

- 5 slices of bacon
- 2 cups yellow onion, diced
- 2 cloves garlic, minced
- 1 cup carrots, diced
- 1 cup celery, diced
- 6 cups chicken stock
- ½ cup orzo
- 1 ½ teaspoons sea salt
- ½ teaspoon fresh ground pepper
- Parsley, fresh, chopped to taste

Directions:

Cook bacon in pan over medium-high heat until crisp. Place bacon on plate lined with paper towels. Save 2 tablespoons of fat from pan. Add the garlic, celery, carrots, onions to the pan with a pinch of salt. Cook the veggies over medium heat for several minutes, stirring periodically. Place chicken breasts in Crock-Pot and cover with veggies and chicken stock. Cover and cook over LOW heat for 5 hours. Halfway through cooking time, take out chicken, shred it up, and then place back in Crock-Pot along with orzo. Garnish each bowl of soup with diced bacon and fresh parsley. Serve hot.

Nutritional Values:

Calories: 507, Total Fat: 7 g, Saturated Fat: 1 g, Sodium: 220 mg, Carbs: 87 g, Fiber:

23 g, Sugars: 10 g, Protein: 28.3 g

Sweet Potato Black Bean Chili

Total Cooking Time: 6 hours 35 minutes

Servings: 6 (3/4 cup per serving)

Ingredients:

Chili:

- 1 medium yellow onion, diced (+coconut or olive oil)
- 3 medium sweet potatoes, scrubbed and rinsed, in bite-size pieces, 4 cups
- 1 16-ounce jar salsa, chunky
- 1 15-ounce can black beans with salt
- 2 cups vegetable stock, + 2 cups of water

Optional Spices:

- 1 tablespoon chili powder
- 2 teaspoons cumin, ground
- ½ teaspoon cinnamon, ground
- 1-2 teaspoons hot sauce

For Toppings (optional):

- Fresh cilantro
- Chopped red onion
- Avocado
- Lime juice

Directions:

In a large pan, heat 1 tablespoon of oil on medium heat; add sweet onions, along with salt and pepper. Stir and cook until translucent, about 15 minutes. Add sweet potatoes and cook until potatoes begin to soften, about 20 minutes. Add all ingredients to Crock-Pot and stir; cover and cook on LOW for 6 hours. Serve hot.

Nutritional Values:

Calories: 213, Total Fat: 6 g, Saturated Fat: 0 g, Sodium: 611 mg, Carbs: 47 g, Fiber: 9.1 g, Sugars: 4.4 g, Protein: 6.8 g

Creamy Potato Soup

Total Cooking Time: 6 hours

Servings: 8

Ingredients:

- 1 30-ounce bag frozen hash-brown potatoes
- 2 cans-14-ounce chicken broth
- 1 10.75-ounce can cream of chicken soup
- ½ cup chopped onion
- ¼ teaspoon black pepper, ground
- 1 8-ounce package cream cheese, softened
- Optional toppings: bacon, sliced green onions, cheese

Directions:

In a Crock-Pot, place chicken broth, soup, onion, pepper, and potatoes. Cover and cook on LOW for 6 hours. Add the cream cheese about 30 minutes before soup is done and stir well. Top soup with bacon, sliced green onion, and cheese if you desire.

Nutritional Values:

Calories: 240, Total Fat: 9.2 g, Saturated Fat: 4.6 g, Sodium: 508 mg, Carbs: 27.9 g

Fiber: 1.4 g, Sugars: 1 g, Protein: 7.8 g

Crock-Pot Chicken Parmesan Soup

Total Cooking Time: 7 hours

Servings: 4

Ingredients:

- 1 green bell pepper, chopped
- 4 garlic cloves, minced
- ½ medium white onion, chopped
- 1 can (14.5-ounces) crushed tomatoes
- ½ lb. chicken breasts, raw, boneless, skinless
- 5 cups chicken broth
- ½ cup Parmesan cheese, shredded
- 2 tablespoons basil, fresh, chopped
- 2 teaspoons oregano, fresh, chopped
- 1 teaspoon sea salt
- ½ teaspoon black pepper
- ¼ teaspoon red pepper flakes
- 4-ounces (uncooked) dry penne pasta
- 2 tablespoons unsalted butter
- Chopped parsley for garnish

Directions:

In a Crock-Pot, stir together bell pepper, onion, tomatoes, garlic, chicken, broth, ½ cup cheese, basil, oregano, salt, black pepper, and red pepper flakes. Cover and cook on LOW for 7 hours. Remove chicken about six hours into cooking time and shred it up on a cutting board, then add it back to Crock-Pot, along with penne pasta. Resume cooking. Serve garnished with parsley and Parmesan cheese.

Nutritional Values:

Calories: 247, Total Fat: 7.3 g, Saturated Fat: 3.5 g, Sodium 378 mg, Carbs: 23 g,

Fiber: 4.8 g, Sugars: 5.1 g, Protein: 22.5 g

Crock-Pot Veggie Tortilla Soup

Total Cooking Time: 8 hours

Servings: 6

Ingredients:

- 1 medium onion, diced
- 1 tablespoon olive oil
- 2 medium cloves, garlic, minced
- ½ medium jalapeno pepper, seeded and diced
- 1 (14.5-ounce) can black beans, drained and rinsed
- 1 cup fresh or frozen corn kernels
- 6 cups vegetable broth
- 2 teaspoons chili powder
- 1 teaspoon cumin, ground
- 1 bay leaf
- ½ teaspoon sea salt
- ½ teaspoon black pepper
- ½ teaspoon coriander, ground

Crispy Tortilla Strips: Preheat oven to 400°Fahrenheit. Using a pizza cutter, cut corn tortillas into ½-inch strips. Spread the strips in a single layer on cookie sheet and bake for 12 minutes.

Directions:

In a pan, cook onion and garlic in oil for about 7 minutes over medium heat, then add them to Crock-Pot. Add tomatoes, jalapeno peppers, black beans, corn, broth, cumin, chili powder, bay leaf, salt and pepper to Crock-Pot. Cover and cook on LOW for 8 hours.

Nutritional Values:

Calories: 289, Total Fat: 3.6 g, Saturated Fat: 1 g, Carbs: 53.7 g, Fiber: 11 g, Sugars:

4.7 g, Proteins: 13.8 g

"Pumpkin Pie" with Almond Meal

Total Cooking Time: 3 hours and 15 minutes

Servings: 8 (2.8 ounces per serving)

Ingredients:

- 4 tablespoons coconut oil
- 1 ¾ cups almond meal
- 2 cups pure pumpkin
- 1 teaspoon pumpkin pie spice
- Natural sweetener of your choice, to taste
- 3 eggs
- ½ teaspoon of cloves, ground
- 1 ¼ teaspoon baking powder
- 1 ¼ teaspoon baking soda
- 1 teaspoon cinnamon, ground
- Sea salt to taste

*Directions:*In a mixing bowl, beat together coconut oil and sweetener of your choice. Add eggs and whisk until well combined. Add the pumpkin and spices, almond flour, baking powder, baking soda and sea salt. Pour batter into a greased baking dish and place it in Crock-Pot. Cover with lid and cook on HIGH for 3 hours. When ready, let it cool down and serve.

*Nutritional Values:*Calories: 233.2, Total Fat: 17.36 g, Saturated Fat: 7.15 g, Cholesterol: 69.75 mg, Sodium: 354.61 mg, Potassium: 237.81 mg, Total Carbohydrates: 9.41 g, Sugar: 6.59 g, Protein: 6.6 g

Crock-Pot Citrus Cake

Total Cooking Time: *6 hours*

Servings: *10 (4.3 ounces per serving)*

Ingredients:

- ½ teaspoon orange rind, grated
- ½ cup almond flour
- 1 ½ tablespoons lemon rind, grated
- 1 tablespoon grapefruit juice (freshly squeezed)
- 1 ½ cup almond milk
- 1 cup sweetener
- 1 cup butter, softened
- 4 egg whites
- 3 egg yolks
- 3 tablespoons lime juice (freshly squeezed)

Directions:

In a bowl, beat sweetener and butter. Mix in flour and stir until well blended. Add the lime, lemon, and orange rinds and all citrus juices. Whisk egg yolks and milk in another bowl; pour into bowl with flour mixture and stir well. In a separate bowl, beat egg whites until they form stiff peaks, then fold into the batter; stir. Spoon the mixture into a lightly greased heat-proof bowl/dish and cover with foil. Pour a cup of water into Crock-Pot and place the batter dish into it. Cover and cook on LOW for 5-6 hours.

Nutrition Values:

Calories: 269.63, Total Fat: 20.5 g, Saturated Fat: 12.6 g, Cholesterol: 105.77 mg, Potassium: 102.9 mg, Total Carbohydrates: 18.23 g, Fiber: 0.08 g, Sugar: 16.01 g, Protein: 4.08 g

Crock-Pot Coconut Cake

Total Cooking Time: 1 hour and 50 minutes

Servings: 8 (4.8 ounces per serving)

Ingredients:

- ½ cup butter
- ½ cup coconut oil
- 2 ¼ cup coconut flour
- ½ cup coconut milk
- 1 cup sweetener
- 3 eggs
- 1 teaspoon baking powder
- Dash of salt

Directions:

In a large mixing bowl, mix butter, coconut oil, and sweetener. Add eggs, one at a time, and stir well after each addition. Mix together the flour, salt, and baking powder in another bowl. Gradually add the coconut milk; combine with the butter mixture until it is well mixed. Grease ceramic cooker with butter in Crock-Pot and line with baking paper. Spread dough evenly on baking paper. Cover with lid, and put a few layers of kitchen paper on the lid to absorb moisture. Cook on HIGH for about 1 to 1 ½ hours. When ready, open the lid and take out the ceramic cooker. Let it cool for about 10 minutes. Carefully remove the cake from mold and let it cool for about 1 hour. Serve.

Nutritional Values:

Calories: 308.58, Total Fat: 30.17 g, Saturated Fat: 22.55 g, Cholesterol: 100.25 mg, Sodium: 161.81 mg, Potassium: 233.16 mg, Total Carbohydrates: 8.32 g, Fiber: 0.74 g, Sugar: 6.08 g, Protein: 3.32 g

Walnuts and Almond Muffins

Total Cooking Time: 1 hour and 10 minutes

Servings: 8 (2.5 ounces per serving)

Ingredients:

- ½ cup flaxseed
- 1 cup almond flour
- ¾ cup walnuts, chopped
- 2 eggs
- ½ cup coconut oil
- ¼ cup sweetener
- 2 teaspoon vanilla extract
- ½ teaspoon baking soda
- ¼ teaspoon liquid Stevia

Directions:

Add all ingredients to a mixing bowl and beat until well mixed. Spoon batter into silicone muffin pans. Sprinkle with finely chopped walnuts. Place inside the Crock-Pot, right on the ceramic bottom. Close the lid and cook for about 1 hour on HIGH. Serve hot or cold.

Nutrition Values:

Calories: 384, Total Fat: 35.03 g, Saturated Fat: 13.9 g, Cholesterol: 46.5 mg, Sodium: 100.16 mg, Potassium: 269.16 mg, Total Carbohydrates: 12.88 g, Fiber: 5.26 g, Sugar: 5.72 g, Protein: 8.76 g

Wild Rice Almond Cream

Total Cooking Time: 3 hours and 5 minutes

Servings: 4 (7.2 ounces per serving)

Ingredients:

- 3 cups of almond milk
- ¾ cup wild rice
- 1 cup water
- 4 tablespoons sweetener
- 1 teaspoon butter
- 1 tablespoon vanilla extract

Directions:

Rinse the rice a few times with tap water and drain. Pour all ingredients into Crock-Pot. Close the lid and boil on HIGH for 2 ½ to 3 hours. Stir every 30 minutes. Ladle rice into serving dishes and allow it to cool before serving.

Nutritional Values:

Calories: 126.54, Total Fat: 1.29 g, Saturated Fat: 0.65 g, Cholesterol: 2.54 mg, Sodium: 6.08 mg, Potassium: 134.4 mg, Total Carbohydrates: 23.27 g, Fiber: 1.86 g, Sugar: 1.51 g, Protein: 4.44 g

Crispy Sweet Potatoes with Paprika

Total Cooking Time: **4 hours and 45 minutes**

Servings: **4 (3.2 ounces per serving)**

Ingredients:

- 2 medium sweet potatoes
- 2 tablespoons olive oil
- 1 teaspoon Cayenne pepper, optional
- 1 tablespoon nutritional yeast, optional
- Sea salt

Directions:

Wash and peel the sweet potatoes. Slice them into wedges. In a bowl, mix the potatoes with the other ingredients. Grease the bottom of Crock-Pot and place the sweet potato wedges in it. Cover and cook on LOW for 4- 4 ½ hours. Serve hot.

Nutritional Values:

Calories: 120.72, Total Fat: 7.02 g, Saturated Fat: 0.98 g, Cholesterol: 0 mg, Sodium: 37.07 mg, Potassium: 260.14 mg, Total Carbohydrates: 9.06 g, Fiber: 2.57 g, Sugar: 2.9 g

Lemony Artichokes

Total Cooking Time: 4 hours and 10 minutes

Servings: 4 (5.2 ounces per serving)

Ingredients:

- 4 artichokes
- 2 tablespoons coconut butter, melted
- 3 tablespoons lemon juice
- 1 teaspoon sea salt
- Ground black pepper to taste

Directions:

Wash the artichokes. Pull off the outermost leaves until you get to the lighter yellow leaves. Cut off the top third or so of the artichokes. Trim the bottom of the stems. Place in Crock-Pot. Mix together lemon juice, salt, and melted coconut butter and pour over artichokes. Cover and cook on LOW for 6-8 hours or on HIGH for 3-4 hours. Serve.

Nutritional Values:

Calories: 113.58, Total Fat: 5.98 g, Saturated Fat: 3.7 g, Cholesterol: 15.27 mg, Sodium: 702.59 mg, Potassium: 487.2 mg, Total Carbohydrates: 8.25 g, Fiber: 6.95 g, Sugar: 1.56 g, Protein: 4.29 g

Almond Buns

Total Cooking Time: **20 minutes**

Servings: **6 (1.9 ounces per serving)**

Ingredients:

- 3 cups almond flour
- 5 tablespoons butter
- 1 ½ teaspoons sweetener of your choice (optional)
- 2 eggs
- 1 ½ teaspoons baking powder

Directions:

In a mixing bowl, combine the dry ingredients. In another bowl, whisk the eggs. Add melted butter to mixture and mix well. Divide almond mixture equally into 6 parts. Grease the bottom of Crock-Pot and place in 6 almond buns. Cover and cook on HIGH for 2 to 2 ½ hours or LOW for 4 to 4 ½ hours. Serve hot.

Nutritional Values:

Calories: 219.35, Total Fat: 20.7 g, Saturated Fat: 7.32 g, Cholesterol: 87.44 mg, Sodium: 150.31 mg, Potassium: 145.55 mg, Total Carbohydrates: 4.59 g, Fiber: 1.8 g, Sugar: 1.6 g, Protein: 6.09 g

Almond, Zucchini, Parmesan Snack

Total Cooking Time: **1 hour and 40 minutes**

Servings: **6 (5.1 ounces per serving)**

Ingredients:

- 3 eggs, organic
- 2 zucchinis, thinly sliced
- 1 cup almonds, ground
- 1 cup Parmesan cheese, grated
- Salt and pepper to taste
- Olive oil
- 1 teaspoon oregano
- 1 cup almond flour

Directions:

Wash, clean, and slice the zucchini. Salt and set aside on a paper towel. On a plate, combine Parmesan cheese, almonds, oregano, salt, and pepper and set aside. On another shallow plate, spread the almond flour. In a bowl, beat eggs with salt and pepper. Start by dipping zucchini rounds in flour, dip in the eggs, then dredge in almond mixture, pressing on them to coat. Pour olive oil in Crock-Pot and add the zucchini slices; cover and cook for 1 ½ hours on HIGH. Serve hot.

Nutritional Values:

Calories: 303.33, Total Fat: 24.22 g, Saturated Fat: 3.61 g, Cholesterol: 78.01 mg, Sodium: 160.81 mg, Potassium: 494.68 mg, Total Carbohydrates: 11.09 g, Fiber: 5.23 g, Sugar: 3.62 g, Protein: 14.65 g

Roasted Parmesan Green Beans

Total Cooking Time: 4 hours and 5 minutes

Servings: 8 (4.4 ounces per serving)

Ingredients:

- 2 lbs. green beans, fresh, trimmed
- 2 tablespoons olive oil
- 1 teaspoon salt and black pepper
- ½ cup Parmesan cheese, grated

Directions:

Rinse and pat dry green beans with paper towel. Drizzle with olive oil and sprinkle with salt and pepper. Using your fingers coat the beans evenly with olive oil and spread them out do not overlap them. Place green beans in greased Crock-Pot. Sprinkle with Parmesan cheese. Cover and cook on HIGH for 3-4 hours. Serve.

Nutritional Values:

Calories: 91.93, Total Fat: 5.41 g, Saturated Fat: 1.6 g, Cholesterol: 5.5 mg, Sodium: 337.43 mg, Potassium: 247.12 mg, Total Carbohydrates: 6.16 g, Fiber: 3.06 g, Sugar: 3.75 g, Protein: 4.48 g

Wild Rice Pilaf

Total Cooking Time: *3 hours and 10 minutes*

Servings: *8 (6.8 ounces per serving)*

Ingredients:

- 2 green onion, chopped
- 2 cups long grain wild rice
- 1 cup whole tomatoes, sliced
- 1 teaspoon seasonings, thyme, basil, rosemary
- 4 cups water
- 1 lemon rind, finely grated
- 4 tablespoons olive oil
- Sea salt and fresh cracked pepper to taste

Directions:

Place all the ingredients in Crock-Pot except the seasonings and lemon rind, and give it a good stir. Close the lid and cook on HIGH for 1 ½ hours or on LOW for 3 hours. After done cooking add seasoning to taste. Sprinkle with lemon rind and serve hot.

Nutritional Values:

Calories: 209.81, Total Fat: 7.31 g, Saturated Fat: 1.01 g, Cholesterol: 0 mg, Sodium: 8.69 mg, Potassium: 237.85 mg, Fiber: 2.87 g, Sugar: 1.75 g, Protein: 6.22 g

White Cheese & Green Chilies Dip

Total Cooking Time: *55 minutes*

Servings: *8 (4 ounces per serving)*

Ingredients:

- 1 lb. white cheddar, cut into cubes
- 1 cup cream cheese
- 2 tablespoons butter, salted
- 1 can (11 oz.) green chilies, drained
- 1 tablespoons pepper flakes, (optional)
- 3 tablespoons milk
- 3 tablespoons water

Directions:

Cut chilies into quarters. Place all the ingredients (except milk and water) in Crock-Pot. Close the lid and cook on HIGH for 30 minutes. Stir the mixture until it is well combined and then add water and milk; continue to stir until it reaches desired consistency. Close lid and cook for another 20 minutes. Let cool and serve.

Nutritional Values:

Calories: 173.76, Total Fat: 15.16 g, Saturated Fat: 7.53 g, Cholesterol: 37.71 g, Sodium: 394.08 mg, Potassium: 309.15 mg, Total Carbohydrates: 6.67 g, Fiber: 0.52 g, Sugar: 2.13 g, Protein: 2.88 g

Spaghetti Squash

Total Cooking Time: 6 hours

Servings: 6 (6.8 ounces)

Ingredients:

- 1 spaghetti squash (vegetable spaghetti)
- 4 tablespoon olive oil
- 1 ¾ cups water
- Sea salt

Directions:

Slice the squash in half lengthwise and scoop out the seeds. Drizzle the halves with olive oil and season with sea salt. Place the squash in Crock-Pot and add the water. Close the lid and cook on LOW for 4-6 hours. Remove the squash and allow it to cool for about 30 minutes. Use a fork to scrape out spaghetti squash.

Nutritional Values:

Calories: 130.59, Total Fat: 9.11 g, Saturated Fat: 1.27 g, Cholesterol: 0 mg, Sodium: 6.79 mg, Potassium: 399.95 mg, Total Carbohydrates: 13.26 g, Fiber: 2.27 g, Sugar: 2.49 g, Protein: 1.13 g

Piquant Mushrooms

Total Cooking Time: Low Setting-4 hours or High-2 hours

Servings: 3 (13.2 ounces per serving)

Ingredients:

- 2 tablespoons ghee/butter
- 1 lb. mushrooms, fresh
- Ginger, grated
- 1 onion, chopped
- 2 cloves garlic, chopped
- 1 tablespoon olive oil
- 1 teaspoon chili powder
- Basil, oregano, parsley, and thyme, to taste
- 2 cups water
- Salt and pepper to taste
- 1 tablespoon fresh lemon juice

Directions:

Rinse and slice mushrooms. Peel and grate ginger. Place mushrooms and all remaining ingredients in Crock-Pot. Stir in the water. Cover with lid and cook on LOW for 3-4 hours or on HIGH for 1-2 hours. Just before serving, sprinkle with fresh lemon juice and parsley. Serve with steak bites.

Nutrition Values:

Calories: 95.01 , Total Fat: 5.17 g, Saturated Fat: 0.75 g, Cholesterol: 0 mg, Sodium: 21.7 mg, Potassium: 563.92 mg, Total Carbohydrates: 7.97 g, Fiber: 2.42 g, Sugar: 4.9 g, Protein: 5.33 g

Artichoke & Spinach Mash

Total Cooking Time: 2 hours and 25 minutes

Servings: 8 (5.6 ounces per serving)

Ingredients:

- 1 ½ cups frozen spinach, thawed
- 2 cans artichoke hearts, drained and chopped
- 1 cup sour cream
- ¾ cup Parmesan cheese, freshly grated
- ½ cup Feta cheese, crumbled
- 1 cup cream cheese
- 2 green onions, diced
- 2 cloves garlic, minced
- ¼ teaspoon ground pepper

Directions:

Add artichoke hearts, spinach, and other ingredients to Crock-Pot. Stir until all ingredients are well combined. Top with cream cheese. Cover and cook on LOW for 2 hours and 15 minutes. Before serving, give dish a good stir.

Nutrition Values:

Calories: 258.99, Total Fat: 20.42 g, Saturated Fat: 11.93 g, Cholesterol: 63.44 mg,

Sodium: 436.59 mg, Potassium: 394.51 mg, Total Carbohydrates: 8.45 g

Fiber: 4.07 g, Sugar: 2.53 g, Protein: 10 g

CPSIA information can be obtained
at www.ICGtesting.com
Printed in the USA
LVHW020204180723
752756LV00014B/875

9 781952 832086